Anonymous

Pocket dictionary of Spanish technical terms

Salzwasser

Anonymous

Pocket dictionary of Spanish technical terms

1. Auflage | ISBN: 978-3-84605-376-8

Erscheinungsort: Frankfurt, Deutschland

Erscheinungsjahr: 2020

Salzwasser Verlag GmbH

Reprint of the original, first published in 1869.

POCKET DICTIONARY

OF

Spanish Technical Terms,

COMPRISING ALSO

THE MOST USUAL FRENCH AND PORTUGUESE

TRADE NAMES,

AND FORMING A COMPLETE LIST OF ALL GOODS ORDERED
THROUGH BIRMINGHAM HOUSES, FOR SPAIN
AND ITS COLONIES, MEXICO, CENTRAL
AND SOUTH AMERICA.

BIRMINGHAM:

CHARLES REDFERN, OLD COURT HOUSE, HIGH STREET.

———

MDCCCLXIX.

PREFACE.

THIS Pocket Dictionary is intended to supply Merchants with the means of interpreting all orders from Spain and its Colonies, Mexico, and Central and South America. The Author, during many years, has acted as translator of these orders, for various houses; and the present little Guide includes the technical terms for all articles ordered for the above-named markets, directly or indirectly from Birmingham establishments, that have come within his extensive experience. He can confidently affirm, therefore, that it embodies the correct translation of the technical terms employed by correspondents in these different countries, and that it will, in consequence, be found invaluable and indispensable in all merchants' offices. Besides, it will serve as a complete list of goods for exportation, usually ordered from Birmingham, by London, Liverpool, and Manchester houses, for the same markets.

Another thing the author would call attention to, is that no Dictionary gives these Technical Terms, as they are not pure Spanish, but sometimes Indian words rendered into Spanish, and sometimes English, French, German, Italian or Portuguese words under a Spanish adaptation. At the same time the usual French and Portuguese terms employed in Spanish countries, are given, *as used* there, though they are not always pure.

The terms supplied are those used in orders, not that they are correct or pure Spanish, but because they are more or less impure, and can only be known through experience.

For these reasons, the Author assumes that the work will furnish to Merchants a reliable and useful guide for their purposes.

The price may be considered high, but it is on account of the limited number of copies that can possibly be sold, as the work will only commend itself to persons having some relation with countries in which Spanish is the native tongue, however corrupted.

But, notwithstanding the high price, the Author hopes to meet with sufficient encouragement to enable him to publish the whole work, which may run into twenty to twenty-four numbers; and should the sale of the first number warrant it, the whole may be printed within a short time.

DICTIONARY

OF

SPANISH TECHNICAL TERMS.

Abalonas	Beads.
Abalorios menudos	Small beads.
Abanico	Fan, iron gig lamp.
Abecedarios ó cartulinas con sus numeros	Alphabets and numbers.
Abillanador, pā berbique	Almond-shaped bit, brace counter sink bit.
Abolladura	Chased work.
Abotonadores (pā cinchas) de Plata	Slide or half-moon buttons (Lima); belt clasps (Guat.); button hooks.
Abrazadera pā cortina	Curtain bands.
Abrazadores de laton, &c.	Ferrules, brass, &c.
Abridores de latas ò cajas	Tincase openers for sardines, &c.
Abrochadores de algodon	Cotton laces.
Acabado, bien	Perfect, complete, faultless.
Acanaladores pā carpintero	Plough planes.
Acanaladores con sus armazones de madera	Cooper's crosses with wooden handles.
Acanalado	Grooved, furrowed, or corrugated.
Accareto. hilo	Packthread, twine.
Accesorios	Accessories, requisites.
Accion de la compania de gas, &c.	Shares of gas company, &c.
Acciones, galapago con sus	Stirrup leathers (saddle with its).
Aceche, alcaparrosa, caparrosa	Copperas, green vitriol, sulphate of iron.
Aceite de linaza, crudo, quemado	Linseed oil, raw, boiled.
Aceite de higuerita comun, de la India, de castor / Aceite Palma Christi ó recino	Common or Indian castor oil.
Aceite de bacalao ó merluza, de pescado	Cod liver oil, or fish oil.
Aceite de esperma	Sperm oil.
Aceite de olivas, de almendras	Olive or almond oil.
Aceite de ballena	Whale oil.

1

Aceiteras ó aceilatas con sus frascos	Cruet frames with glasses.
Aceiteras pā maquinistas	Oil cans for machinists.
Aceituno	Olive green.
Aceña	Water mill.
Acepilladura	Shavings.
Acequia	Canal or channel.
Acerado, acerino	Steeled, or made of steel.
Acerico, acerillo	Pin cushion, small bolster.
Acero, colado, fundido	Cast steel.
Acero, planchuela, cuadrado, ochavado, de barra	Flat, square, octagon steel, in bars.
Acero dulce pā muelles	Soft spring steel.
Acero ampollado, vejiga, ojo de sapo granito	Blister steel.
Acero de agua	Water steel, finest tool steel.
Acero pā cinceles, pā torno	Turning-tool steel, steel for chisels.
Acero pā calzar	Steel for welding.
Acero pā corses de sôra	Steel for ladies' stays.
Acero calda fino doble tijera	Fine wrought double shear steel.
Acero buena clase, marca O'	Milan steel.
Acero Aleman, Ingles, Suecia	German, English, Swedish steel.
Acerado	Small pack-saddle used for riding.
Acetre	Small water bucket, holy-water pot.
Aciculador	Polisher, burnisher.
Acicate	Long-necked Moorish spur, with rowel.
Aciche	Two-edged tool for tilers, for cutting and adjusting.
Aciche, caparrosa	Copperas.
Acion	Stirrup leather.
Acopada, tornillos cabeza	Screws with wine-glass shaped heads.
Acorozado ò blindado, buque	Iron-plated ship.
Adamascado	Damask (drapery), embossed (bedsteads).
Aderesas,-zos pā cajon de difunto	Coffin furniture.
Aderezado,-sado	Stiffened with dressing.
Adornos pā feretro	Coffin furniture.
Adornos pā cuadros, espejos	Ornaments for pictures or looking-glasses.
Afiladores pā carnicero	Butchers' steels.
Afiadores d'aco pā facas com cabo de ponta de veado (P.)	Steels for table knives, with taper stag handles.
Afiadores d'aco pā facas com cabo de ponta com rodas (P.)	Steels for table knives, with wheels.
Agallas pā tinta	Gall nuts.
Agallonadas, cucharas	(Spoons), a raised fluted pattern, braided.
Agarraderas-res pā cortinas	Handles, curtain bands.
Agarraderas pā cartas, pā comodas	Letter clips, commode handles.
Agarraderas pā baul, pā alzar	Trunk or lifting handles.

Agarraderas pã cajon de difunto	Coffin handles.
Agarraderas de 2 chapitas pã bualitos	Trunk handles with two small plates.
Argamasa	Derby cement.
A granel	In bulk.
Agrimensor, cadenas de	Land surveyor's chain.
Agrinches, aguindes, aguinches, tacises,-sas	Tacises, calabozo matchets.
Agrio ò fuerte, alambre de metal	Hard or unannealed brass wire.
Agua fuerte	Aquafortis.
Aguamaniles con sus requisitos	Toilet sets with their fittings.
Aguarras	Turpentine.
Agujas de arreo	Harness or packing needles, or muleteers'.
Agujas fucates	Bolt-rope needles.
Agujas pã coser, de taladro	Best drilled-eyed sewing needles.
Agujas de enfardelar, taladrar ò de 2 filos	Packing needles (or with two edges.)
Agujas de tiza, pã bordar, chapel, de tambor	Long embroidery needles, (marked with chalk).
Agujas pã talabartero	Saddlers' needles.
Agujas pã coser velas	Sail needles.
Agujas pã empaquetar, empacar, coser faldas	Packing needles.
Agujas pã hacer medias	Knitting needles.
Agujas con ojo de plata	Silver-eyed needles.
Agujas de la reina	Queen's needles.
Agujas de grabado	Etching needles.
Agujas de cataratas	Couching needles.
Agujas de mechar	Larding pins.
Agujas ojo redondo sin canal	Round eyed needles without furrow.
Agujas gambutas	Real drilled-eyed blunts.
Agujas mediana	Betweens (needles).
Agujas pã maquina	Machine needles.
Agujas largas pã coser	Long sewing needles.
Agujas pã colchones	Needles for mattresses.
Agujas de jarreta	Bodkins.
Agujas pã pucheras	Needles for making collars.
Agujas compoteras	Compoteras needles.
Agujerado, agujereado planchuela	Drilled or perforated flat iron.
Agujereadores	Punches.
Aguijones acero pã bueyes	Ox-goads.
Ahoyadores pã café	Coffee diggers.
Aisladores pã telegrafo	Isolators for electric telegraph.
Ajuar de laton pã hombre solo	Brass set for one man, consisting of brass bedstead, 6 chairs, small round table, a console, and 2 arm chairs.
Ajuar de casa	All the furniture of a house.
Ajustar, sierra de	Adjusting saw.

Alacena, aldabitas pā	Cupboard hooks and eyes (or small pantry).
Alacran, bagueta de pistola con	Swivel (pistol ramrod, with).
Alambre pā ligaduras	Wire for ligatures.
Alambre pā cerco	Fencing wire.
Alambre hierro, acero, cobre, metal laton	Wire of iron, steel, copper, brass.
Alambre, cobrizado, de pelo	Wire, silk-covered, as thin as a hair, for artificial flowers.
Alambique	Stills for distilling.
Alvânças (P.)	Handspikes.
Albaces	Executor, executrix.
Albarda, albardon, albardilla	Pack-saddle, saddle.
Albaca	Manilla lamp.
Albayalde	White lead, paint, also zinc.
Albeitar	Farrier.
Alcanfor	Camphor.
Alcaparrosa verde	Green copperas.
Alcarrana, cerraduras completas con	Plate or box in door cheek.
Alcarrazas	Dresden covered vases.
Alcarrazas de barro	Porous or unglazed water-bottles, pitchers or jars.
Alcayatas hierro ordinarias	Iron hooked spikes or hooks, common.
Alcayatas pā tuberia, laton con espiga	Pipe hooks, looking-glass supports.
Alcayatas machihembradas hierro dulce	Wrought iron hook-and-eye hinges.
Alcayatas hierro concha de metal pā espejo	Spikes or hooks for looking-glasses, screws with brass shell head.
Alcayatas y bisagras	Hook-and-eye hinges.
Alcayatas pā los carriles	Railway spikes.
Alcayatas metal con espiga pā, clavar, pā cuadros	Brass hook, with spike to drive, for pictures.
Alcayatas pā ventana	Window stays.
Alcayaticas de hierro	Hook-and-eye hinges.
Alcazas de cobre, alcuzilla	Copper oil cans, cruet stand.
Alcoba, alcobilla, alcobita	Alcove, bedroom.
Alcohol, alcol	Alcohol, antimony, black-lead.
Alcotana	Pick-axe.
Alcrebite, azufre	Sulphur, brimstone.
Alcribis	Small tube at back of forge, through which runs pipe of bellows.
Aldabas, pā puertas, de espiga	Hasps, door hasps, spiked hasps.
Aldabas de metal pā reten	Brass cabin hooks.
Aldabas de reten con el gonce cerrado, harponeado	Cabin hooks with spike, closed and jagged.
Aldabas hierro pā postigo	Half-door hasps, shutter.
Aldabas de reten	Stay bars, hasps and staples, brass cabin hooks.
Aldabas hierro con sus hembras	Hook-and-eye hinges.

4

Aldabas laton pā cajones de comoda, aparadores y mesa	Brass handles for commode drawers, drawers and tables.
Aldabas de reten charolades de espiga ó chapa	Japanned iron door hasps with spike or plate.
Aldabas pā ventanas	Stays for windows.
Aldabas de patente	Registered shutter bars.
Aldadas hierro sobre chapa	Door fasteners on plate
Aldabas con grampas pā ventanas	Hasps and staples for windows.
Aldabas con estribos	Hasps and staples with snipe.
Aldabillas,-villas	Hooks and eyes for one or two-leaf doors.
Aldabillas de chapa de laton con sus pitones	
Aldabillas de varilla de laton	Cabin hooks.
Aldabillas de hierro pā postigo	Iron hasps for one-leaf doors.
Aldabillas metal pā escaparate	Cupboard hooks and eyes, or hasps.
Aldabillas de gozne con sus pitones	Hooks and eyes with snipe.
Aldabillas de laton ó hierro con sus hembrillas de rosca pā armarios	Brass or iron cupboard hooks and eyes with screws.
Aldabillas de sosten	Iron shutter-latches.
Aldabillas pā alacena de 2 caras	Double-faced iron cupboard hooks and eyes.
Aldabillas metal con sus hembras	Hooks and eyes.
Aldabillas hierro fundido con sus hembrillas ó ganchos	Cast iron bed-hooks and eyes polished on both sides
Aldabillas ó ganchos de metal con hembrillas	Brass bed-hooks and eyes, both sides polished.
Aldabitas de metal	{ Brass hooks and eyes for door hasps { Small brass cabin hooks and eyes.
Aldabon con chapa pā puerta	Door-plate hasps.
Aldrabas,-vas (P.)	Door hasps.
Alemanisco, adamascado	Sing damask (applied to cloth made in Germany).
Alemanisco de algodon	Cotton alemanisco, coloured cotton table covers.
Alefris	Mortise ; hole cut into wood.
Alesnas pā clavar finas	Fine pegging awls.
Alesnas pā puntar, puntear	Stitching awls.
Alesnas pā aperar	Stabbing awls.
Alesnas pā taco	Awls for nailing the heel.
Alesnas arqueadas, derechas	Bent, straight awls.
Alesnas emplantillar	Sewing awls.
Alesnas cuadradas á bridir	Harness awls.
Alfabeto, candados de	Letter padlocks.
Alfange	Hanger or cutlass, large hanger.
Alfardas (cuchillos)	Carpenters' drawing knives.
Alfileres clavadores	Pricking pins.
Alfinetes de lataô, ferro (P.)	Brass or iron pins.
Alfileres grandes sacaniaga	Large blanket pins.
Alfileres de patente con guarda de seguridad.	Patent safety pins.

Alfileres cabeza enteriza	Solid head pins
Alfileres dorados	Gilt pins.
Alfileres canastilla	Baby pins.
Alfiletero	Pincase.
Alfombra	Carpet, carpeting, woollen rug.
Alforja	Saddle-bag.
Algebena (P.)	An earthen jug.
Algodon	Cotton.
Alguaza (P.)	Hinge.
Algibe,-jibe, cubos de	Well buckets, cistern.
Algallardas, de hierro con sus machos	Stay bars with staples
Alguidaces	Pans to wash vegetables in.
Alicates	Nippers, pincers, pliers.
Alicates pulidos boca chata	Bright flat nose pliers.
Alicates, corte al lado	Side cut pliers.
Alicates, ponta chata e redonda (P.)	Round and flat nose pliers.
Alicates de cortar (P.)	Pliers or pincers to cut.
Alimentador, lamparitas con	Lamps with feeders
Alisadores (peines)	Plain short combs, imitation tortoise.
Alistar	To make ready.
Almagre,-gra	Spanish brown.
Almas de cañamo, cadenas alambre con	Wire rope with inside of hemp.
Almadanas	Best bright - faced hammers for breaking mineral, or (La Union) light masons' hammers.
Almidonados, royales	Starched or stiff royals.
Almireces bronce con sus manos Almofariezas de lataô (P.)	Brass mortars and pestles.
Almofacas reforçadas, 6 pentes (P.)	Strong 6-bar currycombs.
Almofarizes de bronze (ferro) (P.)	Brass or iron mortars and pestles.
Almohadilla	Pincushion, small bolster or pillow
Almohazas	Currycombs
Aloodes (P.)	Californian picks
Alpaca pã vestido de sôra	Alpaca for ladies' dresses.
Alpaca negra labrada ó lisa	Alpaca, figured or plain for linings, mixed cotton and wool.
Alpaca ò alpana, Bandejas de	German silver (Barcelona) trays.
Alquireces hierro fundido, pã boquillas de fuelles	Tue irons for mouths of bellows.
Alquiribis pã fragua	Tues for blacksmiths' bellows, irons for a forge.
Alquitran	Tar.
Alumbre en polvo.	Alum in power.
Alvaiade peneirado (P.)	White lead in powder.
Alviões (P.)	Mattocks.
Alzas	Rifle sights.
Amarillo, canario, cromo, guta	Yellow, canary, chrome, gamboge.
Amarillo ocre, oro	Yellow, gold or ochre.

Amarradas con cordel	Tied with cords.
Amoldadas, copas	Pressed goblets.
Amorces pour fusils (F.)	Percussion caps for guns.
Ampolleta ó reloj de arena	Hour or sand glass, or log glass.
Ampolleta de segundos, media hora, enterizas	Glass for seconds, half-hour, hour.
Ampolleta de angarillas	Glasses of cruet stands.
Ampolleta pã guisar huevos	Glasses to boil eggs.
Anafe hierro charolado	Japanned Dutch stoves
Anafe giratoria	Japanned Dutch stoves with revolving plate.
Anafe copas ó copillas pã candela	Charcoal pans.
Ancinhos reforçadas, 12 dientes (P.)	Strong rakes, 12 teeth.
Anclas pã lanchas con cepo de hierro	Boat anchors with iron stock.
Anclote de caña corte y las uñas grandes	Kedge anchor with short bar and large claws.
Ancres, jas en fer (F.)	Iron stock anchors.
Anca de rana (cerraduras)	Vice hasp locks.
Anca recta (cerraduras con)	Straight hasp locks.
Angarillas, armazones de 5 y 6 ampolletas	Cruet frames with 5 or 6 glasses.
Anillos	Finger rings.
Anillos pã ejes	Axle rings.
Anillos de concesion pã cadena	Connecting links for chains.
Anillos ó roscas pã prisiones de pies	Leg locks with keys.
Anillos pa servilletes de mesa	Table napkin rings.
Anillos hierro dulce, rosca interior	Wrought iron sockets with inside iron screw.
Anis	Aniseed.
Anteojos, de larga vista	Spy-glass or telescope.
Anteojos, pã miopes, de aumento	Spectacles, for short sight, convex,
Anteojos con orejada y numerado en los cristales	Spectacles with spring, and numbered on the glasses
Anteojos de puño	Eye glasses.
Anteojos pã mulas	Mule winkers.
Anteojeros	Horse blinkers.
Antenallas ó tornillos de mano	Hand vices.
Antepechos	Small window balconies.
Antiparas pã el sol	Eye protectors or goggles.
Anzôes azulados (P.)	Blued fish hooks.
Anzuelos pã pescar	Fish hooks.
Anzuelos pã pescar gruesos	Fish hooks for sharks.
Anzuelos torcidos	Fish hooks, best steel bent.
Añil en terroncitos	Indigo in cakes.
Apagador, lampara con	Extinguisher, lamp with.
Aparato pã medir bases de precision	Apparatus for measuring bases with precision.
Aparato de taladrar con brazos	Boring machine with arms, or ratchet brace.
Aparato de alzar trozos	Apparatus to lift trunks of trees.

Aparato pā caballo	Horse trappings.
Aparato de gas completo	Gas apparatus with all the pipes.
Aparato receptor	Receiving apparatus (electric telegraph).
Aparejo real	Blocks and pulleys.
Aparejo pā sospender	Patent lifting apparatus.
Aparejo ó garruchos fuertes con cordel pā levantar madera	Pulleys with rope for lifting timber.
Apariencia, de mucha	Very showy.
Aperar, escoplos pā	Chisels for cutting iron.
Aperos, galapago con sus	Saddle, with all its requisites.
Aplomado, trencilla	Lead colour or drab braid.
Apodaderas	Pruning knives.
Apretadores de tonalero	Coopers' drivers.
Aprecio	Appraisement.
Aradillas hierro fundido	Cast iron bars and bearers.
Arado	Plough and ploughshare.
Arandela pā carreta, pā pernos	Washers for waggons, for a bolt.
Arandela de metal	Brass candle socket.
Arandela de vidrio	Glass candle socket.
Arandelitas	Small iron washers.
Araña pā gas—cristal, metal, bronceado	Gas chandelier, glass, brass, bronzed.
Arcallatas	Hook and eye hinges.
Arcos pā violin	Violin bows
Arcos de hierro (or aró) pā pipa de rom	Iron hoops or, hoop iron for pipes of rum.
Arcos, camas con	Arch, bedstead with
Arenillas, arenilleros	Sand boxes.
Ardoises encadrées pour ecolier (F.)	Framed scholars' slates.
Argallas pā hacer tinta	Nut galls for making ink.
Argolas de lataô (P.)	Brass lasso rings.
Argolas de prata Inglesa galvanizado (P.)	Electro-plated lasso rings.
Argollas pā bueyes ó cochinos	Ox or pig rings.
Argollas con chapa	Rings with plate.
Argollas pā espejo	Rings for looking-glasses.
Argollas con tornillos pā marcos	Rings with screws, for picture frames.
Argollas pā servilleta,-es	Rings for table napkins.
Argollas hierro pā candado	Pad lock rings.
Argoilas pā caballeriza	Stable rings.
Argollas de tornillo giratorio pā amarrar cochinos ó bueyes	Swivel ox or pig rings.
Argollas hierro sin arponear	Iron rings, not jagged.
Argollas metal pā cuadros con tornillo	Brass picture rings with screw.
Argollas hierro con espiga pā candados comunes	Japanned iron padlock rings with spike.
Argollas con espiga de tuerca	Rings with spike for nut for gig shafts.

Argollas sin espiga pā toldo, de toldo	Awning rings without spike.
Argollas de prision pā pie	Leg locks.
Argollas pā pesebre	Manger rings.
Argollas pā armarios	Rings for wardrobes.
Argollas pā cincha	Lasso rings.
Argollas de tornillo, con chapa	Screw rings, rings with plate.
Argollas pā enchapados	Plate rings for pad locks for trunks.
Argollas grafladas (P.)	Jagged spike rings.
Argollas laton pā cortinas, corniza	Brass curtain or cornice rings.
Argollas de madera pā cortinas, &c.	Wood curtain or cornice rings.
Argollas estañadas de hierro	Tinned iron rings.
Armaduras pā pantallas (P.)	Brass holders for shades.
Armario	Bookshelf, cupboard, wardrobe.
Armazones pā silla	Frames for saddles or saddle-trees.
Armazones de ballena pā paraguas	Whalebone frames for umbrellas.
Armazones.	Furniture in general.
Armellas, candados de cerrojo con	Alcove pad locks with staples.
Armellas ó armillas	Staples for bolts.
Armellas pā laminas (P.)	Rings with plate for screws.
Armellinhas pāra cortinas (P.)	Curtain rings.
Armorrones,-marrones de pipas	Pipe hooks
Arnes pā carro	Cart harness.
Aroladores (P.)	Rollers or winders-up.
Aros pā baules	Hoops for trunks.
Arpeos	Grapnel irons, grappling irons.
Arpilleria pā embalar algodon en rama	Packing cloth for raw cotton, jute bagging.
Arpon	Harpoon.
Arponeada, espiga	Jagged spike.
Arqueria	Arched work.
Arquitrabes	Girders for arch.
Arrame de ferro, lataō (P.)	Iron or brass wire.
Arreos	Set of harness.
Arrejadas pā varas	Ploughshares or paddles.
Arrengados pā mosquetero	Stuffs for mosquito curtains.
Arrimages y carruages	Lighterage and cartages.
Arroba	25lbs. (32lbs. Brazil.)
Arroz redondo bajo	Cheap round rice.
Arroz poco partido	Little broken rice.
Arroz canillitas	Long grain rice (Patna.)
Arroz semilla ó redondo	Seed or round grain rice, (Rangoon)
Arzon, pistolas de	Holster pistols.
Asa, pā puerta	Bow handle, door handle.
Asa de cañon	Barrel handle.
Asa de gozne movediza	Hinge, fall, or folding handle.
Asa colgante de gozne	Bail or pot handle.
Asadores	Roasting spits or jacks.
Asadores de torno	Revolving spits.
Asafates, azafates	Trays, waiters.
Asargado doble	Twilled (double).

Asentaderas,-dores	Razor strops.
Asentaderas pã planchas	Sad iron stands.
Asentadores con boca de acero pã herreros	Steel-fronted stone-dressers' hammers.
Aserrin	Sawdust.
Asiento liso	Plain seat.
Asiento de viento	Air cushion.
Assiettes plates et creuses (F.)	Plates flat and deep.
Asta, cabo de	Horn handle.
Asta, polvorines de	Horn powder flasks.
Asta de madera, palas con	Shovels with wood handles.
Astil	Beam of balance.
Astillero, ataranga, dique seco	Dry dock.
Atados	Bundles or ties (larger than " mazos.")
Atados de cuentas	String of beads.
Atiesada, manta, dril	Stiffened manta or drill.
Atornillador	Screw driver or turnscrew.
Atravesaño, atrave	Cross piece of a girth.
Atincar	Borax.
Attelles (F.)	Hames.
Avalorios (see abalorios)	
Aventajados (orinales)	Rather large sized or full sized.
Avios, tenazas y demas pã herrar caballos	Pincers and other implements for shoeing horses.
Avios correspondientes	Corresponding appurtenances.
Aza,-s, ferro, lataô pã bahul (P.)	Iron, brass trunk handles.
Azadas bien aceradas, sencillas	Hoes well steeled, light.
Azadas con refuerzo	Ribbed hoes or hoes with rib.
Azadas con ojo suelto	Rivetted hoes.
Azadas de ojo	Eyed hoes.
Azadas pã chapear	Hoes for potatoes.
Azadas, boca de	Mouth of hoe.
Azadas sin mango (Rio)	Hoes without handles, rivetted hoes.
Azadas cambadas	Bent hoes.
Azadas de descepar, de carpir	Grubbing hoes.
Azadas de martillo	Ribbed hammer adzes.
Azadas de cepillos	Hoes and brushes.
Azadas de garganta	Necked hoes.
Azadas reforzadas todas pulidas	Strong patent hoes, all polished.
Azadas aceitadas	Oiled, self-coloured hoes.
Azadones (Guat.)	Hoes.
Azadones, azadas angostas (Mex.)	Narrow hoes or adzes.
Azadones ô houes (Brazil).	Hoes.
Azadones (Caracas)	Grubbing hoes.
Azadones azulados con pito	Blued adzes with plate.
Azadones (Habana)	Ribbed adzes.
Azadones de descepar	Digging hoes, or for pulling up by the root, grubbing hoes.
Azadones de desyerbar	Weeding hoes.
Azadones de martillo	Ribbed hammer adzes.

Azadones sin meHas	Hoes without notches.
Azadones	Pickaxes.
Azadoncitos	Small hoes or spuds.
Azafates de carton charolado, azafatitos	Trays, papier maché japanned, small trays.
Azafran fino de Castilla	Fine Castille saffron.
Azarcaô (P.)	Red lead.
Azarcon en polvo	Red lead in powder.
Azem fino (zinco), folhas de (P.)	Sheets fine zinc.
Azogue, vidrios azogados	Quicksilver, silvered glasses for looking-glasses.
Azoteas, vidrios muy claros pä	Very clear glass panes for roofs of houses.
Azotes de campaña, cabeza martillo	Hammer headed hunting whips.
Azuelas (P.)	Adzes, *say* loop adzes.
Azuelas de costilla	Ribbed adzes.
Azuelas llanas	Flat adzes.
Azuelas media redondas	Half round adzes.
Azuelas gubias *or* gurbias	Bent or hollow adzes (sometimes) hoes.
Azuelas pä calafate de martillo y ojo cuadrado	Square eye hammer adzes for caulking.
Azuelas con su abrazadera	Adzes with bands, or loop adzes.
Azuelas de dos manos ojo redondo	Long hammer adzes (for two hands) round eye.
Azuelas pä carpintero que no tengan martillo agujado por detras	Carpenters' adzes without sharp hammer at back.
Azuelas gubias con estribo y mango pä tonelero	Bent adzes with stirrup and handle for coopers.
Azucarera plateada	Sugar box, plated
Azufre en canuto	Brimstone in stick, sulphur.
Azulado	Blued.
Azul, ultramar, negra, de Prusia, oscuro, claro	Blue, ultramarine, blue black, Prussian, dark, light.
Azul fuerte, pedernal, quemado, prensado (loza)	Flown blue, earthenware.
Azul celeste, bronceado	Sky, bronzed blue.

B.

Bacias de ferro estanhado (P.)	Tinned iron basins.
Bacines, bacinicas, bacenillas	Chair pans, night pans.
Bacinicas con tapas, bacenillas	Chambers with covers.
Bacinicas de afeitar, bacenillas	Barbers' basins.
Badajo	Bell clapper.
Badana	A dressed sheepskin, basil wood.
Badil *or* badila, tenazas, tizonero	Fire shovel, tongs and poker.
Badilejos (Lima)	Masons' trowels.
Bagazo	Cane waste.
Baguecitas pä fusil	Gun cleaning rods.
Bagueta pä pistola con alacran	Pistol rod with swivel.

Bajilla porcelana	China dinner service.
Bajo, verde	Light green.
Bala	Ball, bullet, shot.
Balanças com mostrador redondo, feitio de relogio (P.)	Balances with round indicator, clock shape.
Balance ó saldo	Book or account balance.
Balanzas con platos, platillos, tazas de lata	Beams with tin plate scales.
Balanzas de reloj	Circular balances and scales.
Balanzas circulares de resorte	Spring circular balances.
Balanzas de mostrador	Counter scales or weighing machines.
Balanzas de cruz	Beam scales or balances.
Balanzas de resorte patentes nao relogio, mas de mola y platos de lata, de resorte (P.)	Patent spring balances, not clock shape, but with spring and tin plate scales.
Balastro, masos pā hacer	Mallets or hammers to make road metal.
Balaustres	Staircase railings.
Balbulas de retencion, contencion, (see valvulas)	Stop valves.
Balcones	Balconies.
Baldes hierro galvanizado	Tinned iron buckets.
Baldes folha de ferro estanhado (P.)	Buckets and camp kettles of galvanized sheet iron.
Balines	Shot.
Ballena, cabo de	Whalebone handle.
Balsamo	Balsam.
Bambú caña	Bamboo cane.
Banastas pā carbon	Coal scuttles.
Bancado or banco	Bed or bench.
Banco pā dinero	Bank.
Banco de economia	Savings bank.
Banco filial, sucursal	Branch bank.
Bandas	Flanges.
Bandas rejilla	Netted bandas or waistbands, sashes or scarfs.
Bandas grana	Scarlet bandas, &c.
Bandas ó fajas de burato labrado, carmin ó color tinto	Figured burato, &c., carmine or red.
Bandas pā cortinas	Curtain bands
Bandas de oro (loza)	Gold bands round cups.
Bandas de cuero	Leather banding.
Bandas de gonce pā abrir puertas	Bars to fasten on a door to swing it open.
Bandejas con y sin rebordo	Trays, waiters, (dishes in Guat. and Guay.)
Bandejas con festones	Festooned or flower-bordered trays.
Bandejas floreadas vistosas, los colores bien contradados	Trays with showy flower patterns, colours well contrasted.
Bandejas con entradas	Trays, &c., gothic shape.

Bandejas embutidas con perlas	Trays, &c., pearl inlaid.
Bandejas plateadas	Trays, &c., plated.
Bandejas de folha de ferro envernisadas com ramagem de colores (P.)	Japanned sheet iron trays with flower and leaf ornamentation, various colours.
Bandana (Indianas) colorada	Red bandana, Indianas.
Bandana nacar, tela asargada y color brillante	Turkey red handkerchiefs, twilled, very brilliant colours.
Bañaderas på asiento	Hip baths.
Bañaderas ó tinas	Foot baths.
Baños de cadua	Hip baths.
Baños de chaparron	Shower baths.
Baqueteras de varias piezas på fusil	Cleaning rods of different pieces for guns.
Barandal på los corredores	Balcony railings.
Barandilla en los pies	Foot railings of bedsteads.
Barbadas på frenos, de freno	Curbs or curb chains for bits, for bridles.
Barbadas de cadenilla con ganchos	Curb chains with hooks.
Barbatana em bruto e em pedaços på cabos de rebenques (P.)	Brown cord in pieces for ends of whip lashes.
Baril, pipa, tonel, bocoy	Cask, pipe, hogshead.
Barniz på figurar metal	Varnish or lacquer for giving the appearance of brass to bedsteads.
Barometro de Fortin con "nonis," termometro anexo al aire libre	Fortin's barometer with "nonis" Thermometer annexed, exposed to the open air.
Barrajas	Playing cards.
Barras de hierro	Iron bars.
Barras på estirar	Bedstead tightening bars.
Barras de corrediza	Sliding rods.
Barras de parrilla	Grate bars and bars for bars and bearers.
Barras de hierro templado de sembrar	Well-steeled planting bars.
Barras de resorte	Spring bars.
Barras de coneccion con su compensador de bronce	Connecting bars with brass compensator.
Barras traveseras	Cross bars.
Barras bruñidas taladradas de yarda en yarda	Bright bars drilled from yard to yard.
Barrenas	Augers or gimblets.
Barrenas på berbiques, de punta ó de tres puntas	Bits for braces or centre bits.
Barrenas pasadores	Gimblets.
Barrenas de cuchara or media cuchara	Longpod or shell gimblets or augers.
Barrenas de tornillo	Screw gimblets or augers.
Barrenas espirales	Spiral gimblets or augers.
Barrenas salamonicas caña larga y redonda	Screw eyed augers, long round stem.

Barrenas salamonicas de tillado y ¼ tillado	Twisted augers or gimblets, screw eyed.
Barrenas pā tonelero, pā pipas	Coopers' tap or bung borers.
Barrenas de furo	Ship augers.
Barrenas pā abrir	Machine or double augers.
Barrenitas pā puntillas	Fine gimblets for shoe bills.
Barreranas de cuchara	Shell augers.
Barretas, - itas con lampa y palo (Lima)	Bars with spade and shovel.
Barretas de punta	Iron bars with point.
Barretas de hierro bien aceradas	Well-steeled iron bars (miners').
Barretas de metal	Stair rods of brass.
Barretones (ahoyadores)	Coffee diggers.
Barretones cuadrados pā trapiche	Square bars for sugar mills.
Barrica	Cask, (say) half-hogshead.
Barrillas de cobre pā perno	Copper bars or rods for pins.
Barrillas hierro pā baranda de balcon	Iron rods for balcony railing.
Barrines pā cantero y albañil	Bars for quarrymen and masons.
Barro, loza de	Clay for earthenware.
Barrotes sueltos	Loose bars.
Barrotes pā parrillas	Furnace bars.
Barrujas,-jos	Screw eye augers.
Barrujas (Lima)	Augers.
Barruso de hierro	Rods of round iron.
Bascula	Weigh bridge.
Bascula pā pesar carromates y gateras	Weighing machines for weighing carts and waggons.
Bastidor de rueda pā hacer puntas pā talabartero.	Saddlers' wheel frames.
Bateas	Bowls, tinned iron washing basins.
Bateas (Gibraltar, Barcelona)	Trays, waiters.
Batederas de mezcla	Mortar beaters.
Batedores de (pā) huevos	Egg beaters.
Bateria de cocina, hierro estañado	Tinned iron holloware.
Baticela de cruz (Puerto Rico)	Crupper.
Baul	Trunk.
Bayeta	Bayeta, baize.
Bayeta fajuela	Lancashire or Fajuela baize.
Bayonetas	Bayonets.
Bebedores de pajaros	Drinking cups for birds.
Becerro, becerrillo, pā zapatero	Calf-skin for shoes.
Beches avec manches, (Guat.—F.)	Handled spades.
Bedames, bedanes, bedanos de espiga pā carpintero	Carpenters' mortise chisels, with spike.
Bedames com espiga calçado d'aço (P.)	Steeled mortise chisels, with spike.
Berbiqui con sus barrenas, brocas ó mechas	Boring brace, with bits.
Berbiqui Escoces, berbiquies ó berbiquines con bocados	Coopers' Scottish braces, with bits.
Berbiquies en cartones con 36 barrenas ó mechas	Carpenters' braces on cards, with 36 bits.

Berbiquies pulidos, color de paja	Braces, polished, straw colour.
Bermellon de China, de Holanda	Chinese or Dutch vermilion.
Beta de cañamo	Hempen rope.
Betun pã botas, en pasta, liquido	Blacking for boots, in cake or liquid.
Betun pardo, cerraduras finas	Brown japanned trunk locks.
Bicos de goma pã mamadeira de crianças (P.)	India rubber teats for children's nursing bottles.
Bicheros	Boat hooks.
Bideles, bidiles	Bed pans.
Bigornias,-nes pã tonelero	Coopers' bick irons.
Bigornias de mesa	Bench vice.
Bigornias pã herrero 2 cuernos	Blacksmiths' anvils, 2 bicks.
Billete	Ticket.
Billeteros	Ticket boxes, railway.
Bisagras figura de libro, librillo, listo	Butt hinges.
Bisagras de cancamo, con macho ó machihembradas	Hook and eye hinges.
Bisagras cola de pescado, de pez, de cruceta	Fishtail hinges.
Bisagras cola de pato	Dovetail hinges.
Bisagras de T Escocesas, Españolas de gozne	Scotch tee (or T) hinges, double iron snipe.
Bisagras de rabo y espiga	Hinges, with stay and hook.
Bisagras con arandelas	Hinges with washers.
Bisagras con perno pã poner y quitar las puertas, ó de quit y pon	Hinges with pin, to put on and take off doors.
Bisagras pã frentes de escritorios, de comoda	Hinges for front of escritoir.
Bisagras de porton, de mesa, bisagritas	Inner-door hinges, table hinges, small hinges.
Bisagras, visagras, milagras, misagras (P.)	Hinges.
Bisagras pã encontro (P.)	Back flap, stop butt hinges, to open half, not stiff.
Bisagras grecinhas e desempenadas (P.)	Butt hinges.
Bisagras de carteira (P.)	Desk hinges.
Bitoque	Plug in cocks.
Bitoque	Drill pin of locks.
Blandones de platina de Iglesia	White metal church candlesticks.
Blando ó dulce, metal	Soft or annealed brass.
Blanqueado, cucharas,	Bleached, whitened, spoons boiled white.
Bloques	Blocks, iron, &c., for nailing shoes on.
Blusa suelta	Loose blouse.
Boas pã café	Coffee diggers.
Bobos, cerrojos	Bolts and snipes.
Bocas de fornalla, figura de teja, con sus tapas	Furnace mouths, roof shape, with covers.

Bocas de fuego grandes con su tapa	Large furnace mouths with cover.
Bocados de gonce	Snipe, hinge or jointed bits.
Bocados enterizos	Entire or solid, net jointed bits, or fast mouth.
Bocados de rienda doble con pierna recta	Straight-cheeked bits, for double reins.
Bocados sin correages ó filetes	Bits without leathers or snaffles.
Bocados con escudo de gozne	Bits with bosses and snipes.
Bocados figura de los criollos	Screwed bits with bosses, and half curb chains.
Bocados de gonces con argollas, barbada, escudos, y media luna platinados	Plated swivel bits, with rings, curb, escutcheons, and half moons.
Bocados con argollas y barbada	Bits with rings and curb.
Bocados, sueltos, hateros	Loose mouth bits, Arab bits.
Bocallaves de laton, nacar, &c.	Brass, pearl escutcheons.
Bocallaves pā gaveta	Escutcheons for boxes, &c.
Bocel sencillo	Fluting plane with single iron.
Bocel con gramil	Fluting plane with marking gauge.
Bocel moldura	Moulding plane.
Bocina	Speaking trumpet.
Bocina pā carreta	Wheel hoops or wagon bushes.
Bocoy	Hogshead.
Bojudas de veira (P.)	Chimneys for lamps with flánge.
Bola, boleada	A bowl, curving outwards.
Bolas pā picaportes, &c.	Balls or knobs for latches, doors, beds, &c.
Bolas de hierro taladradas, pā balcones	Iron balls drilled for balconies.
Bolas de billar, pequeñas pā señoras	Billiard balls, small for ladies.
Bolas Otomanes	Ottoman balls.
Bola Inglesa pā botas	English blacking for boots.
Boladera, voladora	Fly wheel.
Boleada, palanganas forma	Wash basins curving outwards.
Bolsa, bolza (pā dinero)	Purse, pocket.
Bolsa de cuero con avios de cirujia	Leather pocket or roll with surgical instruments.
Bolsa pā cazadores	Game bags.
Bomba pā fincas, hierro estañado	Bowls for sugar estates, of tinned iron.
Bomba pā (ó de) batir, de partir	Bowls for stirring sugar, parting bowls.
Bomba con muñones	Bowls with lugs or ears.
Bomba de cobre con cruceta abajo, y cubo reforzado	Bowls, copper, with cross underneath, the socket strong.
Bomba pā relox cristal fino	Fine round glass shade for clock.
Bomba pā lampara	Lamp shade or globe.
Bomba solar, no solar	Solar globes, hemispheres, shades for lamps.
Bomba, candelabra con	Chandelier with water slide.
Bomba de cristal de vidrio	Globe, vase, barrel lamps.

Bomba pā algibe, pozo, de platina pā bul	Well pump, white metal ale machine or pump.
Bomba hierro con piston de cobre y valvulas de bronce	Iron pump, copper rod and brass valves.
Bombas de chapas ò chapa y forzar	Double-action or suction and force pump.
Bombadillas, bombillas de lata de cubo, de vidrio	Tin socket lamps, barrel lamps, glass.
Bombasi de pelo	Printed cloakings. (Guat.)
Bombasil pā forro de zapato	Lamb skin for lining shoes.
Bombilla charolada con tornillo al lado	Japanned socket lamp with screw.
Bombilla pā lamparas de hoja de lata	Tin plate socket lamps.
Bombilla pā maté	Bombillas or tubes for drinking.
Bombones de cubo, de asa, con eje	Socket lamp, counter ale engine.
Bombita, lampara con, (as bombilla)	Kettles for sugar estates with socket, bail handles, cross piece.
Boquillas de metal amarillo pā mecheros	Small feeders for lamps, brass.
Boquillas hierro pā furo	Iron nozzles for funnels.
Boquillas pā sacabocado	Bits for a punch.
Boquillas pā carreta	Bushes, wagon axle bushes.
Boradores	Bits for braces.
Borcelana	Pan stove.
Bordadas, gasas	Embroidered white lappets.
Borde, orinales con borde tendido, ò chato, y redondo	Rim, chambers with flat and round rim.
Borde, cucharon con borde de acero	Ladle with steel rim or flange.
Borde, tachos, tachitos con	Sugar pans with flange.
Borlas de oro, bandas con	Tassels, sashes with gold tassels.
Botas de cordovan, cuero	Leather boots.
Botas de montar	Overalls.
Bote	Boat.
Botes ó potes	Pots for ointment, drums.
Botellas amoldadas, cortadas	Moulded decanters, cut.
Botequin homeopatico	Case for homœopathic medicine.
Botinas	Small boots, ladies' boots, bottines.
Botones pā muebles, de zebra, porcelana, caoba, ebano, laton	Furniture knobs, zebra knobs or buttons, china, mahogany, ebony, brass, &c.
Botones ó tiradores pā puertas	Door knobs.
Botones pā tapacetes, de carruages	Knobs for gig aprons.
Botones con picaportes	Cupboard knob turns.
Botones de perla, nacar, concha, pā camisas	Pearl shirt buttons.
Botones metal blanco pā chaleco	White metal waistcoat buttons.
Botones de metal blanco pā casacas	White metal coat buttons.
Botones dorados grandes	Large gilt coat buttons.
Botones hueso blanco con 4 agujeros	White bone buttons with 4 holes.
Botones de vidrio	Glass buttons.

Botones de seda lisos floreados	Plain, fancy silk buttons.
Botones elasticos pā casaca	Elastic coat buttons.
Botones de metal cascabel	Metal bell buttons.
Botones dorados pā camisas	Gilt metal shirt studs.
Boucles carrées à rouleaux (F.)	Square roller buttons.
Boucles à crampon (F.)	Side loop buckles.
Beucles de trait (F.)	Trace rings.
Bouillotes émaillées (F.)	Enamelled tea kettles.
Boutons jaunes grelots (F.)	Yellow round bell buttons.
Bovedas de cama	Bed tops or canopies
Boya pā buques	Buoy for ships.
Bozal bruñido	Bright head stalls.
Bozal cobre con sus correas cuero	Brass muzzles or bits with leathers.
Brabanta de linho fino en novellas (P.)	Fine hemp pack thread.
Bracenillas ó braserillos pā candela	Brass charcoal pans, burners.
Braguero de via derecha, izquierda	Single truss to right, left.
Braguero de dos vias	Double truss.
Bramante crudo ó brin	Twine, pack thread, packing canvas.
Braseros, braseritos	Charcoal burners.
Braseros ó fogones	Dutch stove, braziers.
Braseiros, de lataô pequenos porta-brasos (P.)	Brass charcoal burners or fire pans.
Brasuli	Line.
Braza	Fathom.
Brazalete	Bracelet.
Brazos	Arms for gas, or brackets.
Brea negrā y rubia	Pitch, black and red.
Bretañas	Bretagnes, (drapery.)
Bretelles (tirantes) pā calzones (F.)	Braces for trousers.
Bridas con bocado redondas y chatas	Bridles round, flat, with bit,
Bridas	Bridles or flanges for joining pipes.
Brides pour chevaux sans mors (F.)	Bridles for horses without the bit.
Bridon	Snaffle bridoon.
Brin de Rusia	Russias, (dry goods.)
Briseras de cristal (palmatenas)	Glass shades, chamber candlesticks, barrel lamps.
Brocas de berbiqui	Bits for braces.
Brocas de manitas	Claw centre bits.
Brocas de cuchara	Shell bits.
Brocas pā zapatero, azuladas, bruñidas	Blued, bright shoe tacks.
Brocado	Brocade.
Brochas surtidas de dos cabiças (P.)	Shoe tacks with two heads.
Brochas redondas pā pintores	Painters' ground brushes
Brochas pā encalar ó dar cal	Whitewashing brushes.
Brochas de paleta pā blanquear, planas pā dar lechada	Whitewashing brushes.
Brochas pā emborrar	Ground white paint brushes.

Brochas pā pintar	Painting brushes.
Brochas de borrar, ponta, traço (P.)	Ground brushes, sash tools, white-wash brushes.
Broches	Clasps and brooches.
Broches pā traje	Hooks and eyes.
Bronce	Brass, *rarely* bronze.
Bronceado	Bronzed.
Brujulas pā faltriquera	Pocket compasses.
Bruñir, limas pā	Files for burnishing.
Bruñido, Bruñidores	Bright, burnishing tools.
Bruto, peso	Gross weight.
Bruzas pā caballos	Horse brushes.
Bruzas de raiz de millo	Dandy brushes.
Budares, buderas, budeles pā casabe ó casada	Cassada plates.
Buceros de vidrio con sus candeleros	Glass candlesticks with sockets.
Bujero de metal, cerradura con	Brass bush lock.
Bujes enterizos	Bush, cotters of axle, bush of lock.
Bul, llaves pā	Pillar engines with stop cocks for bul.
Bullidores anexos a las calderas	Pipes connected with steam boiler.
Burato	Burato, crape.
Burato, pañuelones de burato labrado	Damask crape shawls.
Burenes	Casada plates.
Buriles	Gravers, burins.
Butaca	Arm chair.

C.

Cabadores de hierro	Coffee diggers.
Cabadores de 8 puas pā patatas	Three-pronged potato forks.
Caballetes hierro estañado y galvanizado	Tinned, galvanized iron ridge caps.
Cabeceras, y pieceras	Bed head rails, foot rails.
Cabecitas de plata (Lima.)	Silver ornaments.
Cabestros	Halters.
Cabeza de cardas	Top or frame of cards for carding.
Cabeza avellana, clavos pā forro de buque	Filbert - shaped head, sheathing nails.
Cabeza abultada, clavos	Raised head, rose head nails.
Cabeza pā freno y bocas	Head piece for head and rein.
Cabezadas de suela, cuero, con escudos y frenos	Leather heads and reins.
Cabezadas sencillas	Single head stalls.
Cabezones	Cavesons, nose band for breaking in horses.
Cabezones de hierro charolado con cadenita, con chapa	Japanned iron cavesons with chain, with flap, plate.
Cabilla hierro comun, refino	Round rod iron, common and refined.

Cabilla de cobre	Copper rods.
Cabilla pā buques	Belaying pins.
Cable de lona, de alambre	Hemp, wire cable.
Cabo blanco	Untarred cordage.
Cabo de algodon, de hilo y 4 ramales	Cotton cord, to be of thread, four twist.
Cabo de alambre de metal ó laton retorcido	Twisted brass wire cord.
Cabo pā alesnas de clavar	Nailing awl handle.
Cabo madera sin pintar pā lesnas	Wood awl handle, not painted,
Cabo ciervo ó cuerno de ciervo de ravisa	Taper stag horn handle
Cabo figuritas embutidas, de doble virola	Handle inlaid with small figures, double ferrule.
Cabresoles	Rings for halters.
Cabretilla, platos	Plates, little goat pattern
Cabulleras pā hamaca	Cotton lines.
Cabria	Shears for setting up masts, &c.
Carcerolas de rabo, de 2 asas	Stew pans, long bow handles.
Cacha de venado	Stag horn handle.
Cachimbos	Sugar saucepans.
Cachiporra	Stick with a large knob.
Cacha, peines pā caballo	Horn horse-mane combs.
Cacha, vidrios de, pā linternos	Horn leaf sides of lanterns.
Cacho de cuerno	Horn handle.
Cadenas ó cuerdas de alambre de hierro, con almas de cañamo pā un puente	Iron wire chains or ropes, with interior of hemp for a bridge.
Cadenas metal pā colgar lamparas	Brass chain for hanging lamps.
Cadenas de 2 eslabones pa roscas	Leg chains.
Cadenas de prision pā pezcuezo	Cotters with chains.
Cadenas pa carretas con grampas y tornillos, pā tiraderas de carretas	Wagon trace chains with staples and screw rings.
Cadenas de retranca	Breeching chain.
Cadenas de cadenera, pā tiraderas	Trace chains.
Cadenas de lomo	Back-band chains.
Cadenas de una tira	Chain in one length.
Cadenas de ladera	Side chains.
Cadenas con sus grampas de yugo y pertigo pā carretas con gancho	Chains with staples for yoke and pole, with hook.
Cadenas pā atar bueyes	Chains for fastening oxen.
Cadenas de metal pā quinques	Brass chain for hanging lamps.
Cadenas pā un tiro de una junta de bueyes	Trace chains for a set of oxen.
Cadenas de ramal negras, de eslabon derecho	Negro fetters, straight link.
Cadenas de arrastrar	Drag chains.
Cadenas de oro pā reloj	Gold watch chains.
Cadenas pā garganta	Neck chains.

Cadenas de seda	Silk Chains.
Cadenas sin atrave, 4 grilletas de 15 brazos	Chains without cross pieces, 4 shackles, 15 fathoms.
Cadenas de barbada, cadenita	Curb chains.
Cadenas (F.)	Padlocks.
Café	Coffee.
Cafeteras de plata	Coffee pots, tea pots, (silver.)
Cafeteras de hierro estañado	Tinned iron tea kettles.
Cafeteras con asas movedizas	Tinned iron tea kettles with falling handles.
Cafeteras de cobre de balanza	Swing copper tea kettles.
Cafeteras de maquina	Patent filterers.
Caguama, peinillos de	Imitation tortoiseshell combs.
Caimitos panuelones de, de algodon morados	Caimitos, or common cotton shawls.
Caixas (P.)	Cases.
Caixas de especiarias (P.)	Spice boxes or pepper boxes.
Caja de madera, carton, caoba	Wood, paper, mahogany box, chest, or case.
Caja con herramientas de carpintero	Carpenters' tool chest.
Caja pā labor, pā papeles	Work box, deed box.
Caja de fusil	Gun stock.
Caja de cuchilleria pā señora	Case for ladies' cutlery.
Caja con agujas, forma zapaticos	Small shoe-shaped needle case.
Cajitas con cuchillo y tenedor pā pescado	Cases with fish knife and fork.
Cajitas pā colocar mechas ó pā porta-fosferos	Fusee boxes, cap primers.
Cajitas pā tabaco	Tobacco boxes, snuff boxes.
Cajon, cerraduras de	Till locks.
Cajon de difunto	Coffin.
Cajuelas de tornillos y machos	Screw taps complete.
Cajuelas, pā gaveta	Boxes and plates.
Cajuelas menudas negras	Small black check (drapery)
Cajuelitas majenta	Small magenta check.
Cal hidraulica	Hydraulic lime.
Calabozos de cubo	Socket calabozo matchets
Calabozos Españoles	Bill hooks.
Calabozos con filos por ambos lados	Bill hooks or calabosa matchets, edge both sides.
Calabozos pā albañil	Masons' trowels,
Calamina	Spelter, calamine.
Calcetines de algodon crudo	Brown cotton socks.
Caldeadas y sanas, hachas	Axes, well wrought, without fault.
Caldera con sus accessorios	Boiler with mountings complete.
Caldera ó paila de vapor	Steam boiler.
Caldera y caldero	Kettle or pot, caldera larger pot than caldero
Caldera de lustre blanco	Peru or white lustre bowls.
Calderitas de lata	Camp kettles or small tin plate pans

Calderitos	Small pots.
Caldereteros, caldereros	Coppersmiths.
Calderôes ferro estanhado (P.)	Tinned wrought-iron pots.
Calderos ò fondos hierro fundido	Sugar kettles without feet.
Calderos estañados por dentro	Tinned inside pots, sometimes saucepans.
Calderos sin pies ó sin patas, calderetes	Danish pots.
Calderos con sus tapas y manojos	Pots with covers and loose handles.
Calderos hierro colado con 3 pies	Three-legged cast-iron pots.
Calderos pã evaporar sal	Pans for evaporating salt.
Calderos cobre pã conservas	Copper preserving pans.
Calderos revivificadores	Revivifying iron pots.
Calderos vivificadores pã carbon animal, borde por dentro, con sus tapas	Pots for revivifying animal charcoal with rim or border inside, with covers.
Caldo, cerbeza en	Broth, ale not bottled, in bulk.
Calentaderas	Tea kettles.
Calentadores, de cama	Bed warmers, warming pans.
Calentadores pã hervir agua	Water boilers.
Calentadores de cobre	Copper tea kettles.
Calesa, caleza	Barouche, chaise, &c.
Calesero	Gig driver.
Calibre de bala Española 1 onza, escopeta del	Gun, bore to be for 1-oz. Spanish ball.
Calomelanos	Calomel.
Calzado	Boots and shoes, all kinds.
Calzado, cuchillo	Steeled, knife, &c.
Calzadores	Shoe lifts.
Calzoncillo de punto, de algodon, pã hombres	Men's cotton knit drawers.
Camas chinescas forma de tienda	Tent shaped Chinese bedsteads.
Camas de pabellon y corona	Bedsteads with tent and crown.
Camas de canopia	Canopy bedsteads.
Camas à la Francesa con, sin pabellon	French bedsteads with and without tester.
Camas de medio cielo	Half-tester bedsteads.
Camas sin cielo que se doblen en cuatro	Stretcher bedsteads, no top, 4 fold.
Camas de matrimonio	Matrimonial bedsteads.
Camas de 2 cabeceras ò de cabecera y piecera	Bedsteads with head and foot rails.
Camas con sus pilares y columnas tubulares	Bedsteads with tubular pillars.
Camas de frenos	Beds with bridle bars, branch to which the rings are fastened.
Camafeos	Cameos.
Camandulas ò rosarios de 15 misterios	Rosaries of 15 mysteries.
Cambiavia de 3 carriles	Three-throw (rail) switches.
Cambray del obispo	Bishops' or Victoria lawn.

Cambray de labores encajueladas menuditas	Cambric jaconet, small check patterns.
Cambray pintado	Printed cambric.
Cambray de colores pā enaguas	Camisa lawn, or printed cambric for petticoats.
Cambray de capricho, panuelos de	Cambric handkerchiefs, fancy styles
Cambrona, pana, terciopela	Velvet, cotton.
Camera	Chamber, &c., as of a gun, &c.
Camisas interiores de punto, de lana, de algodon	Knit under-shirts, worsted, cotton.
Camisitas de algodon, de punto, camisetas	Knit white cotton singlets.
Camisitas de seda sin mango	Silk undervests without sleeves.
Camitas	Cots or small beds.
Camon	Felloe.
Campana de Hacienda	Estate bell.
Campana de zaguan	Door bell.
Campana de buzo	Diving bell.
Campanas, codos de 1 ò 2	Elbows for gas with one or two sockets.
Campanillas metal pā bueyes	Tea bells, cattle bells.
Campanilleros	Bell makers,
Campeche	Campechy wood, common logwood.
Canal	Furrow, (cutlery,) groove, gutter.
Canasta	Basket, hamper.
Canasta ò canastro	Large basket, crate of earthenware, &c.
Canastillas pā colgar	Small strainers to hang at the spout of tea pots.
Canastillas labradas de guta percha	Ladies' work baskets.
Canario	Canary colour.
Cancamos	Hook and eye hinges.
Cancarollas com rabo (P.)	Round and flat bottomed pots with long handle.
Cancho ò chancho	Hogskin, India rubber, gutta percha.
Candados, candaditos	Pad locks, small pad locks.
Candados de barra	Alcove pad locks.
Candados de cerrojo con almellas	Alcove pad locks with staples.
Candados de cerrojillo con 2 pestillos	Alcove pad locks with two bolts.
Candados de camara doble	Double tumbler pad locks.
Candados de letras	Letter pad locks.
Candados de talanquera	Dutch pad locks.
Candados de sortija	Ring pad locks.
Candados de viuda	Very commonest pad locks.
Candados de maleta	Portmanteau pad locks.
Candados con guarda de metal, con asa	Pad locks with brass drop, with shackle.
Candaditos	Small pad locks.
Candeados, cadeados, de ferro, lataò patentes (P.)	Iron or brass patent padlocks.
Candeilas (P.)	Boiling-house lamps.

Candelabra con 4 luces	Candelabra with 4 lights
Candeleros de laton torneados.	Turned brass pillar candlesticks.
Candeleros de agujero ancho	Wide socket candlesticks.
Candeleros con guardabrisa	Candlesticks with shades.
Candiles hierro estañado con 2 luces	Sugar estate lamps with 2 lights.
Caneca	Jar.
Caneca de cerbeza	Pint of ale.
Canela picante	Cinnamon, hot.
Caneladores con sus hierros	Plough planes with irons.
Caneladores de tornillo	Screw plough planes.
Caneladores con sus armazones	Mounted planes.
Canella India (P.)	India cinnamon.
Cangierôes de folha de ferro com bico e tampa (P.)	Boxes of tin-plate with cocks and cover, (square outside, rounded inside, to carry liquids on mules' backs.)
Canivetes d'aço, cabos de veado, madreperola, osso, e tartaruga, com folha pã pennas e 1 folha grande feitio de punhal (P.)	Steel pocket knives, handles of stag, mother of pearl, bone, tortoiseshell, blade for pens, and one large dagger-shape blade.
Canillas de cobre pã pipas con platillos	Brass cocks for pipes, barrels, &c., with flange.
Cantara	Water bottle or pitcher.
Cantaros de fierro	Iron pitchers.
Cantaros (Greytown)	Water bottles with screwing-on top.
Cantera, cuñas hierro pã	Quarry wedges.
Cantil (P.)	Plough plane.
Cantina, " loza "	Canteens, five plates with covers.
" Cantis "	Plough planes.
Canto	Edge.
Canto, tira de lona con 2 cantos	Sailcloth girth with 2 selvedges.
Canto de seguridad, Limas tablas gruesas con	Flat bastard files with safe edge.
Cantonera de culata	Butt plate of gun.
Cantonera hierro colado pã puertas	Angle wall guards.
Cantuna negra	Black cantoons.
Canuteros agujas	Needle cases.
Canuteros pã cigarros	Cigar cases.
Canuto, azufre en	Stick brimstone, sulphur.
Cañamazo, agujas pã coser	Needles for sewing canvas.
Cañamo	Hemp, tow.
Cañamo flojo pã coser zapatos	Shoemakers' hemp.
Cañeria hierro dulce, de plomo	Tubing, wrought-iron, lead.
Caño, yardas ò varas de, hierre colado	Tubing, (yards or lengths of) cast-iron.
Cañones, escopeta de 1 ó 2	Barrels, gun of 1 or 2.
Cañoneras pã sillas	Saddle holsters.
Caoba	Mahogany.
Capa, averia, y flete.	Primage, average, and freight.
Capa de señora.	Ladies' cloak.
Capa de goma pã resistir el agua	Waterproof India-rubber Inverness cloak.

Capacetes de papel (P.)	Paper shades.
Caperusas pā quemar piña	Smelting retorts to be used with pine.
Capim, fouces pā cortar (P.)	Sickles to cut grass.
Capotas pā coches	Hoods and aprons for coaches.
Capote hierro galvanizado	Galvanized iron cover.
Capote de goma	Macintosh.
Capuchinas	Tinned hooded snipes, shutter hinges.
Cara	Face or pane.
Caramela	Straw colour.
Carbon de leña	Charcoal.
Carbon de piedra fina	Pure furnace coal.
Carbon pā gas	Gas coal.
Carbon estinto ò coke	Coke.
Carbonera	Coal scuttle.
Cardas de alambure	Wool cards, cards for carding.
Cardemomos	Cardemums.
Cardenillo, verde	Verdegris green.
Carey, carei	Tortoiseshell.
Cargador	Charterer.
Cargador pā fulminantes	Cap chargers.
Carmelita	Carmelita, colour.
Carmesi	Crimson, cochineal powder.
Carmin fino pastillas de	Cakes fine carmine.
Carmin bandas de	Crimson or red bands.
Carpetas (ò neceseres) con avios de afeitar y escribir	Leather cases, with shaving and writing apparatus.
Carpetas papier maché ò albums	Papier mache portfolios or albums.
Carpetas, cerraduras pā	Box locks.
Carreta	Wagon.
Carretages y portes, gastos de	Charges for cartage and porterage.
Carrete de hilo	Spool or reel of thread.
Carrete de algodon blanco	White cotton in reels.
Carreteles hilo	Reels thread.
Carretillas y lanzadores	Reels and shuttles.
Carretillas pā pasta ò maza	Paste jiggers.
Carretillas ò carreton	Hand trucks, cart.
Carretillas pā ruedas	Wheel drags.
Carretoncillo	Wheelbarrow.
Carriles de movimiento	Rails, moveable.
Carrioles	Trundle bedsteads.
Carrisos hilera, de hilo	Spools or reels thread.
Carrisos blancos	White cotton thread on spools.
Carritos de mano 2 ruedas	Hand carts with 2 wheels.
Carro de mula	Cart, mule cart.
Carro con sus arneses correspendientes con movimiento	Carts with harness and rotary movements on axles.
Carromates y gateras	Carts and wagons.
Carruagito carruejito	Perambulators.
Carta	Letter.

Cartabones ó cachitos	Spokeshaves.
Cartabones	Mitre squares, angle bevils, T bevils
Cartabones pā medida pā zapatero	Shoemakers' measuring or size sticks.
Cartabones hierro y madera	Plated squares.
Carteira, fechadura de (P.)	Desk lock.
Carteras, cartesas pā bolsillo	Pocket book.
Carton pā maquinas	Card, mill board.
Cartucheras	Cartridge boxes, pouches.
Cartuchos con postes pā cazar renados	Cartridges with ball for buck shooting.
Cartulinas ò abecedarios con sus numeros	Alphabet and numbers.
Casaca corta de figura levita	Short coat, frock shape.
Casaca larga	Long-tail coat.
Cascabel, bisagras con cascabel	T hinge with joint or roller.
Cascabel gordo, bisagras con	T hinge with stout joint.
Cascabel ò coscoja, hebillas de	Roller buckles.
Cascabel de platina y laton	Dog bells, plated and brass.
Cascanuezes	Nut crackers.
Casco	A cask.
Casimeres, Ingles, apanado	Kerseymeres, English cloth.
Casimeres de union pā pantalones con franjas	Kerseymeres, union, for trousers with stripes.
Caspa (peines)	Dandriff combs.
Casquillos pā la parte angosta de horma	Iron hoops for the narrow part of funnel.
Casquillos, dedales de	Women's thimbles.
Casquillos fierro pā varas	Ferrules for sticks.
Casquillos ó guarnicion pā candeleros.	Sockets for candlesticks.
Cassarolas de folha de ferro estanhado inteiriças (P.)	Entire sheet tinned iron stewpans.
Casseroles à queue (F.)	Long-handle stewpans.
Caticaes de lataô fundido sem aza com mola de os suspender à vella (P.)	Cast brass candlesticks without handle, with spring to raise the candle.
Catre ó cama de arco de 1½ plazas	Bedsteads with arch of 1½ places.
Catre camera de pavellon entero	Tent bedstead.
Catre bronce pabellon entero	Brass bedstead, full tester.
Catre medio pavellon	Brass bedstead, half-tester.
Catre sin pavellon à la francesa	Bedstead without tent, French style.
Catre de toldilla	Tester bedstead.
Catre de tijera, de bolsa	Travelling bedstead.
Catreras	Bed counterpanes.
Cazoleta, cazueleta	Pan of flint lock.
Cazos pā sopa	Soup ladles or tureens.
Cazuelas, comales	Deep, shallow rice bowls.
Cazuelas	Stewpans.
Cazuelas, con asa de fierro	Iron pans with bow handles.
Cebaderas pā escopeta	Brass primers.

Cedazos, cedacitos	Sieves, small sieves or strainers.
Cedazos alambre de hierro ò cerda	Iron wire or hair sieves or strainers
Cedazos alambre reforzados espirales con doble aro	Strong iron wire sieves with double hoop or ring.
Cedro	Cedar wood.
Cejetas gratas	Burnishing instruments, silversmiths.
Celeste mar	Sky blue, celestial, or sea blue
Celosias	Windows, Venetian blinds.
Celosias, tachuelas pā	Venetian blind nails.
Cencerros de composicion pā ganado	Composition cattle bells.
Cendal	Crape.
Cenicero	Ashpan or ashpit.
Cenizas azules	Blue ash.
Centrados, platos	Centered plates.
Ceñidores	Belts.
Cepilleras, loza	Brush trays.
Cepillos, hierros pā, con agujero sin tapa	Smoothing planes, irons for, with hole, without cover.
Cepillos planos (La Union)	Smoothing planes.
Cepillos de vuelta pā curbos grandes	Turning planes for large curves.
Cepillo con su hierro de 3 dientes pā rastillar	Grooving plane with 3 teeth.
Cepillos, de raiz de millo	Brushes, dandy brushes for horses.
Cepillos pā clavar	Card brushes.
Cepillos pā zapatos	Shoe brushes.
Cepillos pā fregar suelos, pā barrer	Scrubbing brushes.
Cepillos pā escaleras	Banister brushes.
Cepillos pā los dientes, ropa, pelo	Tooth, cloth, hair brushes.
Cepillos pā el tocador	Dressing brushes.
Cepillos pā blanquear, de paleta	Whitewash brushes.
Cepillos de redondear	Shoeshaves, spokeshaves.
Cepos hierro pā una pierna, pā zorras	Leg locks for one leg, fox traps.
Cepos de plaina, de rabote ferro com capa (P.)	Smoothing planes, iron, with cap.
Cepos de molduras, differentes ferros (P.)	Moving fillister planes, moulding planes, different irons.
Cepos guilhermes (P.)	Rabbet planes.
Cantil (P.)	Skew plane.
Cera negra	Heel ball, black wax.
Cerbatana	Speaking trumpet.
Cerchas de las camas	Tops of beds.
Cerco, alambre pā	Fencing wire.
Cerdas, gordas	Bristles, stout.
Cerñidores pā azucar	Sugar filters.
Cerradura	Staple.
Cerradura de cerrojo con espiga	Lock with bolt and spike.
Cerradura pā puertas de 1 ò 2 hojas	Single or double leaf-door lock.
Cerradura pā baules con guarda y boquilla	Trunk locks with drop and bush.

Cerradura de dos golpes pā puertas de zaguan	Hall door lock to shoot twice or two-shoot.
Cerradura pā puertas sin pestillo con su contra	Door lock without link, with counterpiece.
Cerradura pā postigo, pestilleras palastras	Single door lock, flat plate door lock.
Cerradura de dos golpes con aldabon y bocallave	Two-shoot locks with knocker and escutcheon.
Cerradura palastra de lacete, de chapa	Plate lock with hasps, plate lock.
Cerradura de aldabon, de aldaba	Lock with hasp.
Cerraduras pā puertas de calles con tiraderas y bocallaves metal	Street door locks with brass chains and escutcheons.
Cerradura de caja de laton pā puertas corredera, pā camarotes	Brass case lock for sliding berth.
Cerradura de cajon de laton surtida de cuqueta escudos y tornillos	Brass case lock assorted, with "Cuqueta" escutcheons and screws.
Cerradura pā puertas de entrada de camara de cajas de laton con sus picaportes	Door lock for entrance of cabins, brass case with latches.
Cerradura guarnicida de laton	Lock with brass bush and furniture.
Cerradura cucajonada sin boton	Case or rim lock, without knob.
Cerradura tripa fuera	Lock with works outside.
Cerradura de mortaja, de embutir	Mortice lock.
Cerradura anca de rana	Vice hasp lock.
Cerradura escaparate, armario con campana	Cupboard lock, with bell.
Cerradura pā carpeta 2 pastillos	Double link box lock.
Cerradura pā gaveta	Drawer or desk lock.
Cerradura pā costurera	Work box lock.
Cerradura pa cajon	Till lock.
Cerradura pā cajuelas, escritorio, pupitre	Lock for small boxes, desks.
Cerradura de molinete con chapas, aldabon llave de cobre pā baules	Trunk lock with plate, back and key of brass.
Cerraduras de baul con armella pā candados	Trunk locks with staple for padlock.
Cerraduras palestres con dos entradas de llave pā cajon y alacena	Plate locks with two entrances for key, for till and cupboard.
Cerrojos	Bolts.
Cerrojos hierro pā puertas	Bright bar alcove locks.
Cerrojos bobos de espiga	Bolts and snipes with spike.
Cerrojos, candados con	Bar padlocks.
Cerrojos y almellas ó almejas, armellas pā puertas	Bolts and staples complete (or with screws to fasten them).
Cerrojos sin cerraduras	Bolts and staples without locks
Cerrojos con gonce	Bolts and staples.
Cerrojos cola de mona	Monkey-tail bolts.
Cerrojos con armellas de espiga pā remaches	Bolts with staples to rivet.

28

Cerrojos, orientales ligeros	Light monkey-tail bolts with brass knob, with up or top plate.
Cerrojos pä frenos	Bridle bolts.
Cerveza blanca, espumosa	Ale, pale, frothy.
Cerveza negra ó porter	Porter.
Cerveza en medios tarros	Porter in stone pints.
Cerveza en tarros enteros ó grandes	Porter in stone quarts.
Cesta	Basket.
Ceston	Large basket.
Cesto pä poner platos	Wicker basket for plates.
Chacaladas, hachas	Axes with sharp edge.
Chagra afilador pä carnicero, zapatero	Steels to sharpen, for butchers, shoemakers, &c.
Chairas, chagras	
Chaleiras de folha de ferro batido (P.)	Wrought sheet iron tea kettles.
Chambel	Fishing line,
Chambetas pä marinero y chambetos	Sailors' knives.
Chamburotes	Screw drivers.
Chancho ò cancho	Hogakin.
Chapas pä hormas	Funnel sheets,
Chapas pä puertas	Finger plates.
Chapas pä baul, puertas, &c.	Trunk, door, &c., locks.
Chapas pa pomos de portas (P.)	Brass rim roses for door lock knobs
Chapetas ó picaportes pä puerta	Door latches.
Chapetas ò manillitas pä ataudes	Gilt handles or plates for coffins.
Chapitas pä baul ò cajon	Small trunk or till locks.
Chaquires de todas colores	Glass beads of all colours.
Chaquetas, betones nacar pä	Pearl buttons for jackets.
Charnela, charnelo pä frenos	Curb chain for bits.
Charreteras	Epaulettes.
Chato, tenazas puntas chatas	Flat, flat-nosed pliers or pincers.
Chaudrons de fer battu, peroles pä pequenas trapiches pä rapadura	Preserving pans of wrought iron, for small sugar mill for waste canes.
Chavetas pä zapatero	Shoemakers' size sticks.
Chaza, chazo, pä tonelero	Coopers' drivers.
Cheveux, pistolets à (F.)	Hair trigger pistols.
Chichara	Rattle for police, or alarum of steam engine.
Chicorras, chicuras	Coffee diggers.
Chicurones	Trenching shovels and spades.
Chifles cobre con cordon pä polvora	Copper powder flasks with cord.
Chifles tarro con cordon pä polvora	Horn powder flasks with cord.
Chillantes colores	Crying, glaring, loud colours.
Chimeneas	Chimneys, patent grates.
Chimeneas pä escopeta, de pistones	Gun nipples.
Chimenes de veira (P.)	Flanged American chimneys.
China, media	China.
Chorizos ò morcillas, maquina pä hacer	Pork sausage or black pudding, machine for making.

Chuchos triples, de triple via, de doble via	Switches (railway,) 8, 2 throw.
Chuchos, corta pluma con tres cuchillos	Pen knife with three small blades
Chulos	Spokeshaves.
Chumaceras	Spindle bearers, pedestals or journey for spindles to work on, row locks.
Chumbo de muniçaô (P.)	Lead shot.
Chuno	Arrowroot.
Chupones de bronce	Brass suckers for pumps.
Churla de canela	Bale of cinnamon.
Ciervo, cabo de	Horn handle.
Cigarreras de cuero	Leather cigar cases.
Cigueñas de fierro pā montar piedras	Grindstones or crank handles, iron windlasses for unloading ships.
Cilindros de fierro	Bars or rods round iron.
Cilindros de planchar	Mangling machines.
Cilindros con sus candeleros	Candlesticks with tulip shades
Cilindros de vidrio con colgantes y candeleros de vidrio	Glass candlesticks and shades.
Cilindros con sus guarniciones de metal	Vase lamps, brass mountings.
Cimiento de hierro ò limadura menuda	Iron cement, small iron filings.
Cimiento superior Romano	Superior Roman cement.
Cinceles pā abrir cajas ò cascos	Chisels for opening cases, casks.
Cincelada	Chased.
Cinchas de lana, estambre	Woollen girths.
Cinchas de 6 cordeles de cañamo	Hemp horse girths, 6 cords each.
Cinchas de piola	Thread girths.
Cinchas de algodon de colores	Coloured cotton girths.
Cinchas	Belts.
Cinta	Ribbon, tape or braid in general.
Cinta blanca de algodon	White cotton tape.
Cinta de costilla	Ribbed or star cotton tape.
Cinta de lana	Worsted or woollen braid.
Cinta pā presillas	Web for boot laces.
Cinta de cuero pā correa	Laces for leather banding.
Cinta pā persianas	Web for Venetian blinds.
Cinta pā medir	Measuring tapes.
Cinta de tinto	Buff leather belt.
Cinta de lana negra labrada	Figured black worsted tape.
Cinta asargado de algodon	Twilled black cotton tape.
Cinzas azules (P.)	Blue ash.
Cios	Finger glasses.
Cirios	Wax tapers.
Cirugia, estuches de	Surgical cases.
Ciseaux pour ongles (F.)	Nail scissors.
Ciseaux à calfat (F.)	Caulking chisels.
Civieres pā el servicio del cabilote	Trollies.

Claraboyas på cubiertos de buques	Dead eyes or deck lights.
Clavazon surtido	Assorted nails.
Claro, café ó azul	Light coffee or blue colour.
Clavaderas, alfileres	Pricking pins.
Clavados, claveteados, cubiertos con cabos	Pinned, rivetted handled knives and forks.
Claviers på botones de chaleco	Waistcoat button fasteners.
Clavitos de cobre på bomba	Copper pump tacks.
Clavos especia	Cloves.
Clavos acopados, cabeza ovalada	Wine glass oval shape headed nails.
Clavos ala de mosca	Fly-wing iron nails.
Clavos ó alcayatas de carril, de alcayata	Railway spikes.
Clavos cabeza bronce figura de concha på espejos	Shell shape brass-headed nails for mirrors.
Clavos cabeza avellana	Copper sheathing nails, filbert-shaped heads.
Clavos på carrilleras	Spikes for rails.
Clavos cobre på forrar ó forro	Copper sheathing nails.
Clavos cortados	Cut nails.
Clavos cabezones	Round head door nails.
Clavos de concha på cuadros	Glass supports, shell nails for pictures.
Clavos på cielos rasos	Rose nails.
Clavos estoperoles, på clavar fuelles	Nails for bellows, scupper nails.
Clavos estaquillas, de punta på zapato	Fine shoe nails.
Clavos de herrar caballos, frisones	Shouldered horse-shoe nails.
Clavos de ramplon på herrar	Caulkin shoeing nails.
Clavos de paleta palmatos punta chata	Flat point nails.
Clavos picados picoteados på llantas	Jagged wagon tyre nails.
Clavos punta afilada	Sharp point nails.
Clavos Romanos de vidrio ó cristal pa cajones	Glass knobs for tills or drawers, curtain pins.
Clavos tillados, ½ tillados	Rose and half-rose nails.
Clavos de tacon	Shoemakers heel tacks.
Clavos hierro batido, colado	Wrought, cast-iron nails.
Clavos punta de trincha, chata ó de paleta	Chisel-pointed, flat-pointed nails.
Clavos con cabeza de laton	Brass-headed nails.
Clavos largos	Railway spikes.
Clavos espiga fina	Sharp-pointed nails.
Clavos de entablar	Rose nails.
Clavos de alambre	Pointes de Paris, wire tacks or nails.
Clavos de cobre fundido på forro de trenes.	Composition sheathing nails.
Clavos på encalabrinar	Spikes, (Mexico) iron rose nails, sharp points.
Clefs de mantelet (F.)	Rim rings.
Cloruro	Bleaching powder.

81

Cloruro de potasa	Chlorate of potass.
Cloruro de cal	Chloride of lime.
Clous à border (F.)	Boat nails.
Clous brouquettes (F.)	Tacks.
Coa	Coffee digger.
Cobadores de hierro sin mango	Unhandled iron coffee diggers.
Cobertores	Counterpanes, blankets.
Cobijas	Corner tiles or gutter tiles.
Cobre, en pasta	Copper, brass, refined copper.
Cobre colorado en laminas pã hacer fondos de salado	Red copper in sheets for the bottom of salting pans.
Cocinas de una olla estañada	Stoves or cambooses with one tinned pot.
Cocinas de fierro	Cooking pots.
Codillos con platillos en una punta cordon en otra	Elbows, flange on one side and screw on the other.
Codillos en el cabo, espumaderas pã ingenio reforzados de cubo con	Strong socket skimmers with small elbow in handle.
Codos de dos bocinas	Elbows with 2 sockets or flanges.
Codos ó varas de boj, enchapados por los cantos	Rules for measuring, with brass edges.
Codos anchos de boj, marfil, ballena	Wide folding rules of box, ivory, whalebone.
Cofaina	Basin.
Cojinetes	Pommel pads.
Cojinetes ò sellas	Railway chairs.
Cokes de cobre	Brass cocks.
Cola, de pez	Glue, isinglass.
Cola de pescado, bisagras	Fish-tail, T hinges.
Coladores hoja de lata	Gravy strainers.
Coladores pã cañon de cafetera	Spout strainers for coffee pots.
Colchas blancas de algodon adamascadas	Counterpanes of white damask cotton.
Colobadas, sillas	Quilted saddles.
Colchetes, colxetes d'arrame de bolonha (P.)	Hooks and eyes, clasps.
Colchon	Mattress.
Coleros, pã engrudo	Glue pots.
Coleta cruda de lino	Brown linen canvas, Hollands.
Coleta pã forro	Flax canvas or Hessian cloth.
Colgaderas de laton (Vera Cruz)	Plate rings for hanging.
Colgadores de ropa	Coat hooks.
Colgadura una	Set of hangings.
Colgadura de laton, de llaves	Brass labels for keys, &c.
Collares pã perros con cadena de eslabon torcido	Dog collars with twisted link chain.
Collares de barbada con cerradura y chapa	Dog collars with lock and plate.
Collares anodinos	Anodyne necklaces.
Collares pã caballos, mulos, con cadenilla	Horse or mule collars, with chains.

Colheres d'aço pā pedriscos (P.)	Masons' trowels.
Colheres de prata Inglesa pā sopa (P.)	Britannia metal soup spoons.
Colheres de prata Inglesa pā chá	Britannia metal tea spoons.
Colheres de ferro estanhado (P.)	Tinned iron spoons.
Colheres de ferro estanhado pā terrina (conchas) (P.)	Tinned iron tureen ladles.
Colheres de ferro estanhado, escumaderas pā cosinha (P.)	Tinned iron kitchen skimmers.
Colleiras de metal grandes pā cacharo (P.)	Large brass dog collars.
Color de romero	Rosemary colour.
Color de carne, medias de seda	Flesh colour silk stockings.
Color natural	Self colour.
Color amarillo, caña bambú	Cane, gold yellow, bamboo yellow.
Color blanco leche	Cream colour.
Color verde manzana	Pea or apple green.
Color azul, celeste, mar	Sky, sea blue.
Color morado, claro	Bright violet.
Color caoba, roble	Mahogany, oak colour.
Colorado	Red.
Colores vivos, seda de	Bright coloured silk.
Colores vivos, muselinas de	Bright colours, muslins of
Columnitas y damas, con sus coronas	Set columns, &c., with their crowns.
Columpios metal con espaldaje de moroco	Brass swing cots or reclining chairs Morocco lined.
Comales	Flat rice bowls.
Combas	Sledge or mixing hammers.
Comboyes	Cruet stands for dinner.
Comedor	Dining room.
Comodas	Chests of drawers.
Compases de regla pā carpintero	Carpenters' rule compasses.
Compases de resorte y tornillo, de calibre.	Callipers.
Compases de resorte y tornillo	Spring and screw compasses
Compases de volta (P.)	Lancashire spring dividers.
Compases con alita, con alientes	Compasses with wing, with rack wing.
Compases de ferro (P.)	Iron compasses.
Compases e tiralinhas de lataô, jogos completos (P.)	Complete sets brass compasses and inking pens.
Compotaras, composteras	Pressed dishes, comports, jelly dishes.
Compuertas pā trenes, ô ingenio	Furnace doors.
Comunes inodoros	Inodorous water-closets.
Concha	Tortoiseshell or mother of pearl.
Concha pā encurtidos, de cabeche	Pickle shell.
Concha de lataô (P.)	Brass scale of balance
Conchadas, planchas	Corrugated sheets.
Condias, cabo de	Mother of pearl handle.

Conduccion à Liverpool	Carriage to Liverpool.
Comutadores	Commutators (electric telegraph).
Conteras metal pā bastones	Brass ferrules for sticks.
Contrapesos pā lamparas	Balance balls or weights for lamps
Contredoré (F.)	White shirting.
Copas amoldadas, cortadas	Pressed, cut glass goblets.
Copas grandes pā vino tinto	Glass goblets for common wine.
Copas pequeñas ó copitas pā vinos generosos	Wine glasses for fine wines.
Copas de vidrio	Bull's eye glass.
Copas metal pā candela, copas ó anafitas pā candela de platina	Brass charcoal or cigar pans.
Copas pā afeitar	Shaving pans.
Copitas ó escudos, frenos con, ó de bocados	Bits with bosses or bridles with bosses.
Copilla metal pā candela	Brass charcoal pan.
Copitas ó escudos de plata (Lima)	Silver bosses.
Copitas pā fosforo	Cap primers.
Copitas pā tomar huevos	Egg cups.
Coples, fosforos de luz en	Boxes, (vestas) matches in boxes.
Coquetier (F.)	Egg cup.
Coquillo	Coquillo cambric.
Coquilla fina sin cola sin cal,	Coquillo cambric, fine without dressing.
Corales pā niños	Children's corals.
Corchetes (Guat.)	Hooks and eyes.
Cordeles pā pescar	Fishing lines.
Cordoncillo de algodon	Chalk lines.
Cordones	Beadings.
Cordovan	Upper shoe leather.
Corona rueda	Cog wheel.
Corona pā tambor de trapiche	Wheel for sugar mill roll.
Corona pā maza	Cog wheel for sugar mill large roller.
Correas, espuelas con	Spurs with leathers.
Correas dobles con sus boquillas pā municion	Double shot belts.
Correas de suela, de cuero	Belting stitched and rivetted at joint.
Correas pā transmision, sopanda de suela	Leather strap or banding for machinery.
Correas de cuero pā maquineria	Leather bands rivetted at joint.
Correages pā maquina, juego de	Set of leather belts for driving machines.
Correages de distintas formas y precios	Accoutrements of different shapes and prices.
Corraderas pā vidriera	Slides for window sashes.
Corredores de buques	Ship brokers (salesmen)
Correias de capotes (P.)	Cloak strap for saddles, thin skin for.
Corredores pā assucar (P.)	Sugar scoops.

Corta alambres	Wire cutters.
Cortadores de azucar	Lump sugar nippers.
Cortadas, copas	Cut goblets.
Corta estaquillas	Peg cutters.
Corta frios, pā plateros	Cold chisels, gravers for silversmiths.
Corta hierros pā abrir cajas	Cold chisels for opening cases.
Corta yerro, escoplo	Chisel for cutting iron.
Corta uñas	Nail scissors.
Corta plumas, de resorte	Pen knives.
Corta plumas y navajas	Pen and pocket knives.
Corte por dentro y por fuera, gubias con el	Inside cut and outside cut gouges
Corte de tijeras, &c., de trinchas &c.	The edge of scissors, &c. ; the cut of chisels, &c.
Corbatas	Cravats.
Corbatines	Neckties.
Corvado, corvo	Bent.
Coscoja	Star wheel of Mameluke bit.
Costales pā envolver azucar	Sugar bags.
Costurera, costurero con pie	Ladies' work box with foot.
Cotanzas	Linen folded in shape of a fan, cotanzas.
Cotellas	Imitation Biscay matchets.
Cotin, fondo blanco	White ground bed ticking.
Coulantes d'attelles (F.)	Slide rings.
Coupè en dedans, en dehors (F.)	Inside, outside cut.
Couplets à charniere, de table (F.)	Butt hinges, table.
Couteaux Indigo, herbes (F.)	Indigo knives, grass knives.
Couteaux avec ferrule à la fin (F.)	Knives with ferrule on the end.
Contellerie de table (F.)	Table cutlery.
Crabadores (P.)	Pegging and stabbing awls.
Crans, scies à crans (F.) ó con maniguetas	Pit saws with tiller boxes and handles (complete).
Cravos de ferrar, cravadores (P.)	Horse shoe nails, shoemakers' awls.
Creas de lino blanco	Bleached linen creas, linen of a middling quality.
Creas á cuadros ó cuadritos	Creas, check and small check pattern.
Creas, imitacion lino	White royals.
Creguela	Creguela (drapery).
Crepano pā horador madera con brocas	Brace with bits to bore wood
Creuse, assiette (F.)	Deep or soup plate.
Oribas de alambre pā albañil y cantero, mas bien finas	Rather fine sieves for masons and quarrymen.
Cribles	Brass wire sieves.
Criel ó maquina del diàblo	Crab or lifting jack.
Crin de Rusia	Russian crin for lining ladies' boots.
Crinolines de esqueleta	Skeleton crinolines.
Crisoles pā fundir bronce, pā fundicion de lapiz plomo	Crucibles of black lead for smelting brass.

Cristales finos	Fine window panes.
Cristales pā el apretador de tela, pā hacer la puntada comun	Crystals for the presser of the cloth for common stitching.
Cristalezadores pā azucar	Sugar crystallizers.
Crochets pour portes à piton, sans patte avec double piton (F.)	Japanned door hooks and stays with snipes.
Crochets pour portes à patte avec piton (F.)	Japanned door hooks on plate.
Crochets à vis (F.)	Screw hooks, lamp hooks.
Crochets et gonds (F.)	Hook and eye hinges.
Crochets avec piton pour fenêtre (F.)	Hasps with staples for windows.
Crochets de mantelet (F.)	Saddle hooks.
Cruzes, balanzas de cruz	Cross for gas fittings, beam scales or balances.
Cruces hierro pā balanzas	Crosses of iron for balances, scale beams.
Crucesitas pā rosario	Small crosses for rosaries.
Crudo, aceite, hilo, algodon	Raw oil, grey or brown thread, unbleached cotton.
Crupones	Crupper covers.
Cruzeta, palas de	Crutch handle shovels.
Cuadradas sueltas	Loose square bars.
Cuadrado, hierro	Square iron or iron bars
Cuadrantes de metal pā sol	Brass sun dials arranged for the meridian.
Cuadros ò carteles con marco	Engravings or show cards in frame.
Cuadros, cuadritos, creas de	Check or small check pattern, as creas.
Cuadrados enchapados	Plated squares.
Cuajado azul	Flown blue.
Cuartas	Nine inches, measure.
Cuartos y listas negras	Black squares and stripes.
Cubiertos de patente, mecanicas pā encuadrinar	Patent binders, mechanical letter and invoice binder.
Cubiertos, cabos claveteados	Common pinned handled knives and forks.
Cubiertos de plata de lata	Tin dish covers.
Cubos de pozo hierro estañado, galvanizado	Tinned iron well buckets, galvanized
Cubos ò potes hierro pā revivificar carbon animal	Cylindrical pots for revivifying animal charcoal.
Cubo	A socket or socket handle.
Cucharas pā albañil remachadas	Masons' trowels, rivetted.
Cucharas ò cucharitas de bruñir, ò cucharillas	Pointing trowels.
Cucharas pā revocar	Plasterers' trowels, masons'.
Cucharas pā mesa ò sopa, pā postres	Table spoons, dessert spoons.
Cucharas pā sal, pā mostaza	Salt, mustard spoons.
Cucharas pā pescado plateadas	Plated knife for fish, or fish slice.
Cucharas de peltre, blancas	Pewter, boiled white, table spoons.

Cucharitas pā café o té	Tea spoons.
Cucharones	Ladles, soup ladles.
Cucharones pā guisado, grandes	Large rice spoons.
Cucharones pā fundicion	Ladles for melting lead.
Cucharones pā carbon, fondos redondos	Coal scoops with round bottoms.
Cucharones ò palas pā recoger dinero, de cobre borde acero	Shovel of copper with steel rim for taking up money.
Cuchilleria	Cutlery.
Cuchillos de pescado	Fishmongers' knives.
Cuchillos pā mallas	Bill hooks, grass pruning knives.
Cuchillos calzados	Steeled knives.
Cuchillos de saladero	Butcher's knives for salting place.
Cuchillos con pomo 3 canales	Knife with 8 furrows, brass caps.
Cuchillos pā maquina de cortar chapas	Cutters for machine for cutting plates.
Cuchillos de redondear, de rascar, pā voltear, de ahondar	Spokeshaves.
Cuchillos de monte, de caza	Hunting knives.
Cuchillos punta de lanza, de punta	Spear-point knives.
Cuchillos punta roma	Round or dub-point knives.
Cuchillos pā ebanista	Cabinet makers' scrapers.
Cuchillos de dos mangos pā quitar marcos	Coopers' shaves to take off marks.
Cuchillos acero pā caoutchouc circulares	Circular knives for India rubber.
Cuchillos pā alfardas	Carpenters' drawing knives.
Cuchillos pā rajar tejamani	Coopers' troes.
Cuchillos cabo de cubo pā cortar las majorcas de cacao	Socket handled knives to cut the ears of cocoa.
Cuchillos pā cortar papel	Paper knives.
Cuchillos pā abrir cajas de lata	Knives for opening tin-plated cases, sardine knives.
Cuchillos punta corva	Curved-point spear knives.
Cuchillos y tenedores ó trinches	Knives and forks.
Cuchillos pā tonelero	Coopers' hollowing, jigger and drawing knives.
Cuchillos pā herradores	Farriers' knives.
Cuchillos pā cortar yerba	Knives for cutting grass.
Cuchillos de trapiche	Sugar mill knives.
Cuchillos pā ingertar	Grafting knives.
Cuchillos pā podar	Pruning knives.
Cuchillos pā picar carne	Mincing knives.
Cuchillos pā carniceros	Butchers' knives.
Cuchillos de doble virola	Waterloo shouldered knives.
Cuchillos con cabo acanalado	Knives with screw handles
Cuchillos chambetas	Sailors' knives.
Cuchillos y tenedores cabo de hueso blanco	White bone-handled table knives and forks.
Cuchillos cabo de ciervo, de hierro	Stag horn, iron handled knives.
Cuchillos de palo colorado	Red handled knives.

Cuchillos pā postres	Dessert knives.
Cuchillones, cachos prieta (P.)	Large knives, black handled.
Cuelga sombreros y paraguero	Hat hooks and umbrella stand.
Cuello	Neck, collar.
Cuentas	Beads, red, blue, white, black.
Cuentas mostacilla	Hail-shot beads, white, black.
Cuerdas pā violin, pā arco, de tripas	Violin bow strings, catgut strings.
Cuerno, polvorines	Horn powder flasks.
Cuero curtido, zurrado	Leather, tanned, curried.
Cuero de concha	Sheets English leather, to be thick or stout, for bands.
Cuero de carnero encharolados	Japanned roans or basils.
Cuero ò suela pā valvulas de bomba	Sheet leather for rims of valves
Cuillers de fer battu étamé, metal blanc (F.)	Wrought-iron tinned spoons.
Cujas (Buenos Ayres)	Bedsteads.
Culibre, marca	Snake mark.
Culibre	Worm of a still.
Culo de acero, dedales plateados	Plated thimbles, steel tops.
Culota plateada	Plated butt end of gun.
Cumbreras hierro galvanizado lisas punta diamante	Diamond point plain galvanized iron ridge caps,
Cuna ò camitas con forro de genero	Cradle with canvas sacking.
Cuna columpio	Rocking cradle.
Cuñas hierro bien aceradas pā rajar madera	Wedges, well steeled, for splitting wood.
Cuñetes	Kegs.
Cuñitas hierro pā carretas	Small iron wedges for wagons.
Curtidos	Pickles.
Cutachas (Mexico)	Horn-handled matchets.
Cutillos	Pruning knives.
Cuvettes de fer étamé (F.)	Tinned iron basins.

D

Dados ò rempujos pā coser, sin armadura	Sailors palms without tops.
Dados y machos, tarrajas con	Screw plate with steel dies for plates.
Dados pā guijos	Plates for shafts, or shaft plates
Dagas con sus vainas	Daggers with sheaths.
Dagas punta de haya	Dagger-point knives.
Damajuanas	Dame Juans or demi-Johns.
Damasco	Damask (drapery.)
Damasco de lana y algodon	Woollen and cotton Damask.
Damasco, loza	Damascus.
Dedaes d'aço pā senora (P)	Ladies' steel thimbles.
Dedaes d'aço pā homem forrados de lataô (P.)	Men's steel thimbles, brass lined
Dedales con guarda	Steel topped thimbles.
Dedos	Fingers (in regard to measurement)
Dejados, cuchillos, bien	Well-finished knives

Delgadas, barritas	Thin, narrow, thin bars.
Delgasador	Distributor.
Demasia de los gastos	Excessive charge of expenses.
Demeloirs (F.), escarmenadores	Dressing combs
Dentadas, hojas de sierra	Teethed saw blades.
Dependiente	Clerk.
Depositos pä aceite	Oil tanks.
Depositos pä agua	Slop jars.
Derechos de dique y municipales	Dock and town dues.
Derrame	Leakage.
Desaguadera pä esponja	Sponge drainer.
Desarmadores	Spanners, wrenches.
Desbarbadores	Welt cutters or rasps.
Descansador, descansadora pä planchas	Sad iron stand.
Descanso	Sad iron stand.
Descascarar el cañamo, maquina de	Hemp-breaking machine.
Deshechos de algodon	Cotton waste.
Deshollinador, desollinador	Turk's head brush, chimney sweep's brush.
Despabiladores, despabiladeras	Snuffers.
Despavesaderas, despavesadores	Snuffers.
Despacho, escritorio	Office.
Desperdicios de algodon pä limpiar maquina	Cotton waste to clean machinery.
Destaquilladores, alesnas	Entering or bookbinders' awls.
Desterronador	Clod crusher.
Destornillador	Coach wrench.
Destornillador pä carpintero	Turnscrews, screwdrivers.
Desviradores	Arvisadores, welt cutters.
Devastadores	Preparatory rolls.
Dias de estadia	Lay days.
Diamante pä cortar vidrios ó cristales, engastado	Diamond, mounted for cutting glass.
Dibujo	Drawing.
Dibujo encendido	Glaring or flaming pattern in drapery.
Dig, dige	Toy.
Dique, seco	Dry dock.
Dique, gastos de	Dock dues.
Dobladas, Indianas	Folded Indianas.
Dobradiça (P.)	Hinge.
Dobradiças pä puertas escareadas ó escariadas	Machine hinges for doors.
Dobradiça de maquina	Machine hinges for doors to lift off.
Dobradiça, fiches estreitos e largos	Dovetail and butt hinge.
Dobradiça detras	Bed and back flap hinge.
Doloirs de tonnelier (F.)	Coopers' adzes.
Dorado	Gilt, lacquered.
Dorados, tanques	Gold lustre mugs.
Douilles (F.)	Sockets.

Draibas ó chazas pā tonelero	Coopers' drivers.
Dril crudo	Unbleached drill.
Dril cazador	Brown linen.
Dril de algodon	Cotton drill.
Dril diagonal de hilo	Diagonal linen drill.
Dril blanco doble labrado	Double white cotton drill, figured.
Dril labrado	Figured drill.
Dril cañamo blanco asargado	White twilled hemp drill.
Dril de hilo pā militares	Linen drill for the military.
Dril crudo cazador	Unbleached linen drill for hunting.
Dril de colores de pintas firmes,	Drill of fast colours.
Dulceras de vidrio medianas	Glass sweetmeat dishes, middle size.
Dulce ó blando, metal	Soft or annealed brass.
Duraderas	Lastings, (drapery.)
Dusias (P.)	Dozens.

E

Ebajadores, empajadores pā tonelero	Coopers' flagging irons.
Ebano	Ebony.
Eclises (F.)	Railway fish bars.
Ecrou (F.)	Nut of table handle.
Ecuerres (F.)	Squares.
Egohines	Hand cross-cut saws.
Ejes de carros	Cart axles.
Ejes con cama y maza ò' muñon, cama	Axles with bed and arm.
Elastico	Elastic web.
Electro plata	Electro-plate.
Emaillé (F.)	Enamelled.
Embalage	Bundling, packing.
Embotellar, llaves de, llave fija y suelta	Bottling cocks, fixed and loose key.
Emboquillas	Bushes for key holes.
Embudo, molinos de, de pasta, de porcelana	Funnel mills, Wedgwood ware hoppers.
Embudo pā colar vino sin rosca	Wine strainer, hopper not to screw on.
Embudo tornillos, cabeza de	Countersunk headed screws.
Embutido de metal	Inlaid with brass.
Embutidores de cuchara ó empajadores	Shell gravers, inlayers.
Embutidores de plateros	Brass stamps for silversmiths.
Embutir	To inlay.
Empajadores pā tonelero	Coopers' flagging irons.
Empaquetar	Packing of any kind.
Empates, pintura blanca de plomo pā	White lead for joints.
Empavonado	Blued.
Enaguaderas	Water bottles or decanters.

Enaguas, enaguillas	Petticoats.
Encabar, lesnas sin	Awls without handles.
Encabas, palas	Handled shovels.
Encabilladores con bola de metal	Bolts or latches with brass knobs in the middle.
Encajes, hilera blanca	White thread lace.
Encajonadas, cerraduras	Rim locks.
Encajuelados, de colores	Intersected pattern, checks, tartan.
Encalabrinar, clavos pā	Rose nails, sharp points, sharp-point spikes.
Encarne, tornillos de	Countersunk iron screws, gimlet point.
Encendido, dibujo	Glaring pattern.
Encerado	Oil cloth tarpauling, (for packing.)
Encontro, bisagras pā (P.)	Brass butt hinges, stop butts.
Encurtidas	Pickles.
Encurtideras ó rabaneras	Pickle or radish shell.
Enfardelar, agujas pā	Packing needles.
Enfriadera pā azucar	Sugar cooler.
Engrudo	Glue.
Enjugatorios	Caraffes and stoppers.
Enloza de porcelana pā pisas	Earthenware flooring tiles.
Embargo	Attachment, embargo.
Embocadura de metal	Brass bush.
Embola	Railway buffer.
Enlozadas, ollas	Enamelled pots.
Enrejado de alambre galvanizado	Iron wove wire or lattice, (galvanized.)
Ensaladeras con pie	Salad dishes with foot.
Ensamblar	To join tubes.
Ensambladores	Rabbet planes.
Ensanchadores pā botas	Boot trees.
Entablar, clavos de	Fine rose nails.
Entalladura	Carved work.
Entenallas de plateria ò platero	Hand vices, silversmiths'.
Enteriza, cabeza de alfileres	Solid head pins.
Entradas en la aduana	Custom house clearance.
Entrefinas	Middle fine.
Envoltario, envuelto	Wrapper.
Envolvidero	Package or truss.
Enverjado	Fences to prevent walkers from spoiling the grass.
Envuelto, hebillas envueltas	Cover, wrapper, covered buckles.
Enxadas (Buenos Ayres) (P.)	Brazil hoes.
Erminettes bleutèes (F.)	Patent blued chisels.
Error de pluma	Clerical error.
Escabadores y escarbadores	Garden rakes.
Escalafadores	Meat hammers.
Escantillones de corredera	Wire gauges, sliding wire gauges.
Escaparate	Cupboard.
Escapolas pā cabidos	Brass hooks.

Escaramales y escamarales	Hoes.
Escarbadores pā jardin	Garden rakes.
Escardillas sin charolar	Field hoes or spuds, (not japanned) thistle spades.
Escarificadores, 12 cuchillos	Scarificators, 12 blades.
Escarlata	Scarlet.
Escarmenadores, peines	Long combs (dressing.)
Escarpas pā abrir cajas, escarpias	Chisels.
Escarpias	Tenter nails with hooked heads, hooks to drive.
Escarpidores, peines de goma	India-rubber dressing combs.
Escarpines	Men's brown socks, also slippers, pumps.
Escobas finas de crin	Fine horse-hair house brushes, or brooms.
Escobas de pared, pā quitar arañas	Turk's head brushes or brooms.
Escobas pā barrer con cabos	Handled sweeping brooms.
Escobas pā lavar el suelo ò pisos	Brooms for washing the floor.
Escobas pā caballos	Horse brushes.
Escobas de cocina	Kitchen brooms or brushes.
Escobenes	Hawser pipes.
Escobillas pā blanquear	Whitewash brushes.
Escobillas pā dientes	Tooth brushes.
Escobillas Irlandesas	Irish or scrubbing brushes.
Escobillas pā empapelar	Paste brushes.
Escobillas pā zapatos	Shoe brushes.
Escobillas pā betun, pā limpiar zapatos	Blacking brushes.
Escobillas pā escalera, balaustres	Stair brushes, banister brushes.
Escobillas pā quitar arañas	Turk's head brooms.
Escobillas pā mesa, redondas	Round table brushes.
Escobillas de mostrador	Counter scrubbing brushes, with 9 rows across.
Escobillas de capricho, caprichosas	Fancy brushes.
Escobillas, de lavatorio, de baño, de cuerpo	Flesh brushes.
Escobillones	Hair brooms, Turk's head brushes,
Escodas	Stone axes or masons' hammers.
Escodas finas pā albañiles	Stone-cutters' hammers, or masons' cutting hammers.
Escodas de 2 bocas de patente	Patent masons' hammers of two mouths.
Escofina pā ebanista	Rasps for cabinet makers.
Escofina pā albeitar	Farriers' rasps.
Escofina de ¼ cana, de 4 caras	Half-round or 4-square files (rasps)
Escopeta fulminante, de fosforo	A percussion gun.
Escopeta de 1 ó 2 canones	Single or double-barreled gun.
Escopeta de viento	Air gun.
Escopeta de baston	Walking-stick gun.
Escoplo de aperar con cabeza de hierro, ò corta yerro	Cold chisel for cutting iron.

Escoplo de aperar	Bricklayer's chisel.
Escoplo de cubo	Socket mortice chisel.
Escoplo de espiga	Firmer mortice chisel.
Escoplo mango hueco	Socket chisel or hollow handled.
Escribanias	Inkstands.
Escribanias de caoba	Mahogany writing desks.
Escritorio	An office, also writing case.
Escuadras de ó para carpintero	Carpenters' squares.
Escuadras madera grandes con hierro y nivel en el extremo	Large wood squares with iron and bevel on the extremity, or ordinary masons' spirit level squares with plumb bobs.
Escuadras falsas ò cartabones	T bevels.
Escudillas	Grecian bowls.
Escudillos (La Guayra)	Hoes.
Escudos pã cama	Bed caps.
Escudos de laton pã tapar tornillos de cama	Escutcheons for covering bed screws.
Escudos de embutir	Escutcheons to inlay.
Escudos pã cabezada	Ornaments on a bit.
Escupideras, de mano	Spittoons, chambers, spitting pots.
Escusado	Water closet.
Eslabon derecho ò torcido de cadena	Straight or twisted link of chain.
Eslabon de lima pã sacar candela, chispa ó pistola	Fire steel with file for striking light.
Esmalto,-e	Enamel.
Esmeril en polvo	Emery in powder.
Esmeril, trigo farina	Emery, fine like wheat flour.
Espadas	Swords.
Espadenes coa puño	Handled furrow matchets.
Espadines pequeños	Small matchets.
Espanadores	Canister brushes.
Esparto	Bass.
Esparragos	Bed poles.
Espatulas, mango de madera	Wood handled spatules.
Espaviladeras	Snuffers.
Espejo, espejitos, cuadro de caoba	Mahogany framed looking glass.
Espejo, sierras de	Saws with looking glass polish.
Espejuelos de oro	Gold spectacles.
Espiga, central	Spike, tang, centre tang.
Espingardas	Muskets.
Espiochas de pico y pala	Patent blued Brazil pick axes, with sharp and flat point or pick, and broad end.
Espiochas pã canteros	Pick axes, Brazil picks.
Espiraus ò estirador	Stretcher or drawer out.
Espolines	Bent and screw neck spurs.
Esponjadas, loza	Sponged.
Esposas de mano	Handcuffs.
Esprimidores de tomate	Tomato drainers.

Espuelas	Spurs.
Espuelas pā calesero	Drivers' spurs.
Espuelas pezcuezo combado, pico corbo	Bent neck spurs.
Espuelas con punta torcida ò pico jorobado	Bent neck spurs.
Espuelas pie de gallo, ò con taloreñas ò de talon	Cock's foot spurs, heel box spurs.
Espuelas hierro estañado con pasador	Tinned iron spur with bolt sawarrows, sinvarrows.
Espuelas con sus correspondientes herrajes y rosetas	Brass spurs with corresponding brass work and rivets.
Espuelas pā clavar ò clavadora, rolletas	Wheel cutters.
Espuelas rectas ó derechas	Straight neck spurs.
Espuelas carcoladas de cuello	Swan neck spurs.
Esperma de ballena	Sperm, spermacetti.
Espumaderas reforzadas pā ingenio	Strong skimmers for sugar estate.
Espumaderas chicas pā tachos (espumadores)	Small skimmers for sugar estate.
Esqueleto, crinolinas de	Skeleton crinolines.
Esquina, esquinero	Corner, angle, corner piece.
Esquinas matadas, cucharas de albañil	Rounded corners, mason's hammersmith.
Esquineros	Angles.
Esquineros metal pā cajitas	Brass corners for boxes.
Esquineros hierro	Angle iron.
Esquineros pā sala	Corner pieces for drawing rooms.
Estacadores pā zapateros	Shoemakers' awls.
Estadia, dias de	Lay days for a ship.
Estambre de lana pā bordear	Yarn for embroidery, fine knitting wool for embroidery.
Estampados, merinos, loza	Printed merinos or earthenware
Estampados lisos, jarros	Plain printed ewers.
Estampados de pajaros	Stamps of birds.
Estañes	Broth bowls or basins, small basins with a cover and plate.
Estañes	Chair pans, stool pans.
Estañado por dentro y por fuera	Tinned inside and out.
Estaño en barrilla, en barritas	Bar tin.
Estaño en panes, en lingote	Block tin.
Estaquilladores	Pegging awls or entering awls.
Estera, cuadros blancos y encarnados	Red and white chequer matting.
Estera de manila pā limpiar los pies	Manilla door mats.
Estearina, candelas	Stearine candles.
Estopa de cañamo torcida altriquinada	Twisted tarred hemp tow.
Estopa blanca hilada pā empaquetar	Spun white tow for packing,
Estiraderas de laton	Brass drawer handles.

Estoperoles	Scupper nails, flat heads.
Estoperoles pā fuelles	Scupper nails for bellows, or bellows nails.
Estoperoles clavos dorados	G. C. chain nails, bellows nails.
Estoperoles pā buque	Deck nails.
Estopillas	Estopillas.
Batiste	Baptiste.
Estraza	Wrapping paper.
Estrella pā espuela	Spur rowel.
Estrevillas, esterillas, estribillas	Shirting, estrivillas.
Estribillos de gozne	Spring bars with hinge plate, stirrups.
Estriados, loza	Fluted.
Estriberas, estriberos	Stirrup leathers.
Estribos, con resorte, estriberas	Stirrups with spring.
Estribos de zapatillos	Slipper stirrups.
Estribos charoladas de campana	Japanned stirrup with swivel.
Estribos y rosetas	Stirrup with slide and rosettes.
Estribos con piso de platina	Gig steps, plated foot gig step.
Estribos pā calesero pā hatero	Driver's stirrups.
Estribos de piso platina pā quitrin	Gig steps plated in the foot.
Estribos, correa pā	Gig steps with leather.
Estribos pā coches con hojas de cerrar	Folding coach steps
Estribos pā correr pā coches	Sliding coach steps.
Estribos de zapato	Heart-shaped stirrups, bottle-eyed stirrups.
Estribos de campana	Stirrups with swivel, bell shape.
Estribos pā volante de vaiven	Moveable gig-eye stirrups.
Estuche de viajar	Travelling case.
Estuche de una ó dos navajas	Case of one or two razors.
Etuche con instrumentos matematicos	Mathematical instrument case.
Estuche suizo de compases	Swiss case of compasses.
Estuche con avios de afeitar	Dressing case complete.
Estuche de herramiento pā carpintero	Carpenters' tool case.
Estufa pā cocina, pā los pies	Iron kitchen range, foot warmer.
Estufa	Stove.
Etamé (F.)	Tinned.
Eteau à main (F.)	Hand vice.
Etiqueta de pergamio	Label.
Etrilles pour cheval, peigne au dos (F.)	Curry combs with mane combs at the back.
Existencias	Stock.
Extractos finos	Fine extracts (for toilet.)

F

Facas	Knives.
Facas de parena (P.)	Vine-knives.
Facas de carnicero (P.)	Butcher's knife.

Factura	Invoice.
Fagoteados, ejes de hierro	Fagotted iron axles.
Faience	Earthenware.
Fajas ó bandas, burato tinto	Deep red burato bands.
Fajas de suela	Leather driving band, band leather.
Fajas (Buenos Ayres)	Diaper web, side-saddle web.
Fajas de hilo	Brown straining web.
Fajuela	Arragonese scarfs, (men's.)
Fajuela ó bayeta	Baize, fajuela.
Falda	Flap of a saddle.
Fallebas de hierro pā puertas con 5 grampas	Chain bolts with 5 staples.
Falsas, escuadras	Slide bevels, false squares.
Familia	Familia, family shirtings.
Fantasie, fantasia	Fancy (drapery)
Fardos	Bales.
Faroles de talco	Horn lanterns.
Faroles de babor y estribor	Larboard and starboard lamps.
Faroles de popa ó mastelero	Poop or top mast lamps.
Faucilles (F.)	Sickles.
Fechaduras pā gavetas (P.)	Till locks.
Fechadurinchas (P.)	Small locks.
Felpa	Iron sheet.
Felpudo de lana	Plush.
Fer feuillard (F.)	Sheet iron.
Fers à repasser (F.)	Sad irons.
Ferrages	Tools.
Ferros pā rebotes	Plane irons (see also *hierros*.)
Fiaira de tarracha, fleira (P.)	Screw plate.
Fichas	Counters or tokens, shilling and sixpence size.
Fieltros de lana	Woollen felts for rollers.
Fierros dobles ò sencillos pā cepillos	Double or single plane irons.
Fierros pā castrar caballo	Irons for gelding horses
Fierros pā torcer soga	Irons for twisting rope
Figuras, de sable ò puñal	Shape, as of a sword or dagger
Filaila, bombasi	Bombasin, bombasette.
Filetes	Snaffles, fillets, as gold fillet round cups.
Filets à (F.)	With fillets or bands, as table forks.
Filets (F.)	Bits.
Filets acier, mors avec (F.)	Bits with steel snaffles.
Filieres (F.)	Screw plates.
Filos por ambos lados, calabozos	Cutting edge both sides
Filos por fuera, por dentro	Cut inside, cut outside.
Firmes colores	Fast colours.
Fisgas ó harpones de 8 puas pā pescar	Harpoons.
Flanela	White flannel serge.
Flechas ó colgadores	Rods and hooks.

ó trensa	Fringe, as of a shawl, drapery.
hierro pā arcos de bocoya ó	Iron hoops for hogsheads or pipes.
	Hoop iron.
de laton, una cara bruñida	Brass hoops, one side polished.
s pa sangrar caballo	Horse fleams.
	Freight.
le romero, color	Rosemary flower or lavender colour.
	Loose.
metal de colores pā cortinas	Enamelled flowered brass curtain pins.
les pā cortinages, mētal pin-	Brass painted curtain pins.
nes de metal pintados	Brass painted curtain pins.
nes de cama, de cortinas	Bed curtain pins.
os	Flower stands or vases.
s pasantes pā calderas de vapor	Interior flues of steamer boilers.
les, pā calentar hierros, de nchar	Dutch stoves.
nes de embutir con sus regillas	Havana stoves with their grates.
les con patas largas	Braziers' stoves with feet.
ó funda con pistolera, gala- o con	Saddle cover with pistol holsters.
	Ground (as in pattern of drapery).
de cobre pā alambique	Copper bottoms or pans, copper still bottoms.
os ó peroles	Cast iron sugar pans or bottoms.
os ó calderos	Sugar kettle without feet.
os ó pailas pā sacar azucar	Bottoms or pans to make sugar.
do, hierro	Wrought iron.
ones de espiga, formones pla- con espiga	Firmer chisels.
ones gurbias con espiga	Firmer gouges.
ones con cubo ó tubo	Socket chisels.
ones pā cortar hierro en frio	Chisels to cut cold iron.
lla	Furnace.
lo	Chafing dish, portable little oven or furnace.
de cobre	Lining, sheathing, cover, sheathing copper.
pā almohada	Pillow cases.
de flejo	Iron sacking of bedsteads.
de lona, entero	Canvas sacking, seamless cloth sacking.
, papel de	Packing paper.
r, clavos pā	Sheathing nails.
ros ó pistones de escopeta, il	Percussion gun caps.
ros de cera, de luz	Wax matches, vestas, lucifers.
ros vivo	Phosphorus.
reras	Nipple wrenches or keys.

Fouets à marteaux (F.)	Hammer whips.
Fracos, frascos på polvora	Powder flasks.
Fragua portatil con fuelle completa	Complete portable forge.
Franela	Flannel.
Frasquera	Bottle case, liqueur case.
Frascos	Glasses of cruet frames.
Frasquitos caledor de tinta	Bottles kalydor, bottles ink.
Freio de meia lengua på caballo	Bits half tongue for ponies
Fresada	A blanket.
Fregatas ó grandes carros de ferro carriles	Large railway waggons.
Frenos angostos de gonce	Narrow bits with jointed mouths.
Frenos de carro, 2 argollas	Cart or mullen bits.
Frenos 4 argollas	Bits with 4 rings.
Frenos con codillo y coscoja	Mameluke bits with spikes and ring.
Frenos con capas	Mameluke bits with rosettes, bits with bosses.
Frenos sin capas	Mameluke bits without rosettes.
Frenos de campo	Camp bits.
Frenos de segunda	Strong Galloway snaffle heads and reins.
Frenos de hierro batido	Wrought-iron bits.
Fresadas, frasadas tintas	Red blankets.
Frioleras en articulos de fantasia	Trifles.
Frisones, clavos	Shouldered horse-shoe nails.
Frontiles y frontis	Front pieces.
Fruteros, fruteras con pie	Fruit dishes with stand or foot.
Fuelles på herrero, herreria	Smith's bellows.
Fuelles på cocina, på casa	Kitchen, house bellows.
Fuente hierro fundido	Cast-iron fountain.
Fuente på pescado, på pastel, pastillo	Fish dish, pastry dish, pie dish.
Fuente på aqua caliente	Dish for hot water.
Fuente llana ò tendida con tapa	Shallow dish with cover.
Fuente honda con tapa	Deep cover dish.
Fuente sin costura, de orilla	Dish without joint or seam, edge dish.
Fuerte ò agrio metal	
Fuete y foete på montar à caballo, på darle á los caballos	Whip for horses.
Fuete con rabisa y martillo	Whip with thong and hammer.
Fulminantes på fusil	Percussion gun caps.
Fulminantes rayadas på escopeta	Ribbed percussion gun caps.
Fundas de cuero	Leather saddle covers.
Fundas de cuero	Pistol holsters.
Fundas de camas	Bed sacking.
Fundo, ojetes con uno ó dos	Eyelets with 1 or 2 rims.
Furadores (P.)	Gimlets.
Furos på hormas	Nozzles for sugar funnels.
Fusil	Gun, generally a military arm.
Fustes de sillas de montar	Saddle trees.

G

Gafas de hierro pä uso de barriles	Hooks for hooking barrels.
Gafas pä el sol	Eye protectors or goggles.
Gafetas	Hooks and eyes.
Galapagos con asiento comodo y todos sus aperos	Saddle with easy seat and all its requisites.
Galapagos cuero de maraño	Hogskin saddles.
Galapagos de estaño	Ingots or pigs of metals.
Galon de seda, oro, plata labrado pä muebles	Lace for furniture, silk, gold, silver lace.
Galvanometros	Galvanometers.
Gamarrones de suela fuerte pä bestias	Head collars.
Gambutas, agujas	Real countersunk drilled eyed blunts
Gamusas pä limpiar coches	Wash leather, or chamois leather for washing coaches.
Ganchitos pä bordar	Crochet hooks.
Ganchos hierro pä postigos	Bed hooks and eyes.
Ganchos pä el pelo	Hair pins.
Ganchos con guardacabos dobles chicos	Ship hooks and thimbles, double and small.
Ganchos de bichero	Boat hooks.
Ganchos con sus florones	Hooks with roses.
Ganchos y redanchos	Ship hooks and thimbles.
Ganchos pä colocar vestidos ò perchas pä ropa	Hat and coat hooks.
Ganchos pä guindar ropa, pä roperas	Hat and coat hooks.
Ganchos pä encimeros	Hooks for backbands.
Ganchos pä bombas	Hooks for lamps.
Ganchos pä calzar botas	Hooks for drawing on boots.
Ganchos pä clavar	Tyne hooks.
Ganchos de hierro	Iron hooks.
Ganchos pä tapa pies	Hooks and rings for carriage aprons.
Ganchos con roscas	Hooks with screws.
Ganchos morunos	Moorish hooks.
Ganchos pä llantas	Tyre hooks.
Gante	Gante, drapery.
Gante, gante lona	Ghent, sail cloth.
Garabatos	Hooks, hat and coat hooks.
Garantizado	Warranted, guaranteed.
Garapin	Grapnel.
Garlopa hierros dobles de haya	Beechwood single-iron trying-plane.
Garlopines	Jack planes.
Garras de ojal	Hide cuttings or clippings.
Garrafas	Bottles or decanters.
Garrancha con florones	Saw pulley with ornaments.
Garrucha de madera	Wood jib block.
Garrucha de hierro pä cama	Iron bed castor.
Garrucha de laton, de rueda	Brass pulley.

Garruchas con cordel, rueda laton	Brass wheel pulleys with rope.
Garruchas de una rueda	Single wheel screw pulleys.
Garruchas de metal con espiga	Brass pulleys with iron spike and screw.
Garruchas con tornillos	Pulleys with screws.
Gasa, estampada	Gasa, printed muslin.
Gasa lisa	Jaconets, plain muslin.
Gasa, de motones	Strap or binding of pulley blocks, (iron.)
Gasa de motones, guardacabos metal pā	Brass thimbles for block straps.
Gasometro pā gas	Gasometer.
Gateras y carromates, maquina pā pesar	Waggons and carts, machine to weigh.
Gatillo	Trigger.
Gatos ò lirones sencillos	Light lifting jacks.
Gavetas, gaveticas, pā purificar azucar	Drawers, small drawers, sugar coolers.
Gemelos, un par de ó gemelos de teatro	Double opera glasses.
Genero de cuerda	Kind of cord (drapery.)
Genero	White book fold familia, shirtings.
Genero de colchon de algodon	Cotton stuff for mattresses.
Genero de lana pā forros	Crimson cloakings.
Geringas de goma elastica	Syringes, elastic glyster pipes.
Geringas de fuente en estuches	Fountain syringes in cases.
Gibes, gives, ò cedazos	Wire sieves.
Girantes, parillas redondas ordinarias	Round revolving enamelled gridiron.
Giratoria, pistola, lampara	Revolving pistol, socket lamp.
Globos de cristal	Glass globes.
Godanhos (P.)	Three-prong potato forks.
Golpe, candados de un	Single-shoot padlocks.
Golpeadores de puerta	Door knockers.
Goma lacre	Gum lac.
Goma laca clara	Shell lac, gum light of colour.
Goma Arabiga	Gum Arabic.
Goma elastica	Elastic, India rubber.
Goma en plancha	India rubber sheet, galvanized.
Goma en plancha pā maquineria	India rubber sheet for machinery.
Goma en tiras redonda y cuadrada pa maquineria	India rubber in lengths, round and square for machines.
Gonces, gonzes, nudos pā puertas	Snipe hinges for doors.
Gonces hierro bruñidos pā escaparate	Bright iron cupboard hooks.
Gonds à pattes (F.)	Snipes, snipe hinge with stay.
Gorditas, lesnas	Rather thick or thickish awls.
Gorras ò morriones	Military caps.
Gorrion, pico de	Spear point.
Gourmettes (F.)	Snaffles.
Grabado (loza)	Engraved.

Grada	Harrow.
Gradillas ó parillas pā ingenio	Bars and bearers.
Gramil con tornillo	Marking gauge with screw.
Gramil, ó gromil	Mortice gauge.
Grampas y espigas abiertas	Open snipes and staples, staples or clips.
Grampas de hierro	Hasps, staples, eyes for bolts.
Grampas con chapa de platilla pā quitrin	Footmen, holders with plate for grates.
Grampas pā pertigo	Shaft or pole staples.
Grampas y argollas pā carreta	Waggon staples and rings.
Grampas de espiga pā sillas	Saddle staples with spike.
Grampitas de espiga	Small spiked staple.
Grana	Cochineal.
Granates en ramo, en racimo	Garnets, in a branch.
Granatorias de peso español	Set of silversmith's weights.
Granel, carbon à	Coal in bulk or loose.
Grano de oro	Grograms, drapery.
Grasa pā ferro carril	Grease.
Gratas de alambre pā plateros	Wire brushes or scratches for silversmiths.
Gratas	Burnishing instruments.
Gratas pā disyerbar pā cafetal	Weeding hoes.
Greda	Chalk.
Grilhas (P.)	Gridirons.
Grilletes con cadena ó empates duras	Shackles or connecting links, with chain.
Grilletes pā dos pies	Fetters for two feet.
Grilletes de cadena pā buque de eslabon derecho de 20 brazos	Shackles of straight link ship chain, chain of 20 fathoms.
Grilletes cadena de 15 brazos	Lengths of chains of 15 fathoms.
Grillos de prision bruñidos pā pie	Bright leg locks.
Grueso, de buen ó un poco grueso	Thick, a good thickness.
Gruperas	Cruppers.
Guadañas con sus mangos correspondientes	Scythes with corresponding handles
Guacal con madera	Wood handled water bowl or wash basins.
Gualdrapa	Saddle cloth or housing.
Guarales pā pescar	Fishing lines.
Guarda de candado	Drop of a padlock.
Guarda brisas	Barrel, ship lamps.
Guarda brisa de mesa	Shade for lamp, table lamp.
Guarda brisa floreada	Indian shades.
Guardacabos, abiertos, cerrados	Ship thimbles, open, close.
Guardacenizas con sus juegos correspondientes	Fenders with sets fire irons.
Guarda fuegos ó resguardos	Fenders.
Guardamonte	Trigger or gun lock guard.
Guardias, papel con	Paper with border, for a house.
Guardillas matizadas	Variegated borders, (drapery.)

Guaridas	Retreating docks.
Guarnicion y cadena, collares cuero con	Leather mule collars with hames and chain.
Guarnicion pā collares	Hames for collars.
Guarnicion de laton	Brass mountings for lamps.
Guarnicion pā resortes de puertas	Brass furniture for door springs.
Guatacas de cubo	Bent socket hoes.
Guayacan	Lignum vitæ.
Gubias ó gurbias de varias figuras y tamaños pā hacer labores en la madera ò tallar	Firmer gouges of different shapes and sizes, for making figuring in wood, and for cutting.
Gubias ½ derechas ½ revesas	Gouges, half straight, half reversed bevel edge.
Gubias revesas de espiga	Reversed bevel edged spike gouges.
Gubias con rebajo por dentro	Gouges with bevel inside.
Gubias de bocamanga	Long gouges.
Gubias de cubo, de Espiga	Socket and firmer chisel gouges.
Gubias pā torneador	Turning gouges.
Guebanozes (P.)	Nut crackers.
Guijos pā mazas chicas	Shafts and centres for small rollers.
Guijos, dados pā	Shafts, plates for.
Guijos con sus trampas, espiga cuadrada	Shafts with centres, square spike.
Guijos pā trapiche	Sugar mill shafts.
Guillames y machihembrados	Rabbet and grooving planes.
Guillames oblicuos, oblicisos	Skew rabbet planes.
Guillamon	Rabbet plane.
Gurupelas, guruperas ó gruperas, bocados con frenos	Bits with bridles and cruppers.

H

Habladeras pā tonelero, y jabladeras	Coopers' crosses.
Hachas Brazileñas	Brazil axes.
Hachas de cuña	Wedge axes.
Hachas de labor ò labor entero	Labor axes.
Hachas de ½ labor	Half-labor axes.
Hachas de tumba	Felling or falling axes, tumba axes.
Hachas pā labrar	Axes for shaping planks or wood, as carpenters use for felling trees.
Hachas pā tejamani, hachitas } Hachas pā tejamani con mangos }	Shingling hatchets, handled
Hachas pā toneleros	Coopers' adzes.
Hachas zuelas, pā carpinteros	Carpenters' axes.
Hachas pā azucar	Sugar axes.
Hachas pā cantero	Stone axes.
Hachas de mano, de Bizcaya	Helved axes.
Hachas pā carniceros	Butchers' choppers.
Hachas pā abordar	Boarding axes.
Haches à abattre (F.)	Felling axes.
Haches trous ronds (F.)	Axes, round eye.
Hachitas tejamani	Small hatchets or gentlemen's shingling.

Hachitas de oreja	Claw hatchets.
Hachitas pā cocina	Kitchen choppers or cleavers.
Hachotes (F.)	Adzes.
Hachotes de couvreurs (F.)	Slaters' hatchets.
Hachuela de mano con uña y de martillo ;,	Hand hatchets with claw and hammer.
Halachas	Plane irons.
Halachas	Pick mattocks or pick axes.
Hamaca	Hammock.
Harasse (F.)	Crate.
Harina, de aro	Flour, arrow root.
Hataca	Pot handle, large kind of wooden ladle, rolling pin.
Hateros, estribos	Driver's stirrups.
Hazuelas	Hammer-head adzes.
Haya	Beech wood.
Hebillas con argollas	Buckles, D buckles and ring.
Hebillas forradas, cubiertas con cuero	Leather covered buckles.
Hebillas metal pā cinturon	Brass belt buckles.
Hebillas pā cartuchero	Cartridge-box buckles.
Hebillas hierro estañado de cascabel con coscoja	Tinned iron roller buckles.
Hebillas pā bridas	Buckles for bridles.
Hebillas pā cinchas	Girth buckles.
Hebillas con sus chareteras pā calesero	Buckles and loops for drivers.
Hebillas pā sombreros	Hat buckles.
Hebillas pā collares	Horse collar buckles.
Hebillones	Belt buckles.
Hechura	Make or shape.
Hembras pā aldavas pā puertas	Eyes for door hasps.
Hembras con roscas	Eyes and screws.
Hembras de tornillo de herrero	The boxes of a smith's vice.
Hembrillas con espiga	Eyes with spike for stay bars, eyes for bolts.
Heniquen, tela pā sacos	Heniquen, canvas for coffee bags.
Herradura, pā pie, pā mano	Iron shoe, hind and fore feet.
Herradura pā caballos, pā mulas, pā bueyes	Horse, mule, ox shoe.
Herrages pā carros	Iron work of railway waggons and carts.
Herramientas pā carpinteros, pā zapateros, pā herreros	Carpenters' shoemakers' and smiths' tools.
Herramientas, dos juegos completos de los que se necesitan pā estaquillar	Two complete sets of awls for boring for pegs, or to fasten pegs with.
Herramientas de carpinteria, herreria, pā zapa	Carpenters,' smiths,' miners' tools.
Herrar, clavos de	Shoeing nails for horses, oxen.
Hierros pā torcer soga	Irons for twisting rope.

Hierros pā cepillos con capa	Plane irons with cap or cover.
Hierros abiertos, fechados	Open or with holes, closed or without holes, irons.
Hierros pā planchas de caja	Irons for box and irons.
Hierros pā calafates	Caulking irons.
Hierro pā hembras de balcones	Iron for the knobs of balconies.
Hierro colado, fundido, de fundicion	Cast iron.
Hierro dulce batido, de paños, forjado	Wrought iron.
Hierro de planchuela, de platina	Flat iron.
Hierro de cabilla redondo	Round rod iron.
Hierro cuadrado	Square iron.
Hierro maleable	Malleable iron.
Hierro cilindrado	Rolled iron.
Hierro angular, esquinero, canalejo	Angle iron.
Hierro en lingotes	Pig iron.
Hierro de cuchillo	Iron for knife blades.
Hierros pā cepillos	Plane irons.
Hierro estañado galvanizado	Tinned galvanized iron.
Hierros de punta pā planchar, pā sastres, pā sombreros	Sharp pointed sad irons for tailors, for hats.
Hierros dobles sencillos	Irons, double or single for all tools.
Hierros pā castrar caballos	Irons for gelding horses.
Hierros de carpinteros, pā caballero, caja de	A gentleman's chest of carpenter's tools.
Hierros pā marcar madera	Timber scribes.
Hierros pā planchar	Sad irons.
Hierros derechos pā cabar tierra	Straight irons for digging earth.
Hierros pā chimenea	Set of fire irons.
Hierro pā flores	Iron for making ornaments or flowers with.
Hierro comun, refino, marca Biscaya	Common, refined, mark Biscay iron.
Hierro angulo ordinario cantos gruesos	Ordinary angle iron with thick edges.
Hierro laminado	Laminated iron, sheet iron.
Hierro laton de hierro, planchas de	Thin sheet iron, sheet iron.
Hiladores	Spinners or spinning mills.
Hilado lavado, de tejer	Washed weaving thread, grey water twist.
Hilaza rosada	Rose colour or pink yarn.
Hilaza cruda	Brown shoe thread.
Hilaza de algodon encarnada	Bright red cotton yarn.
Hilaza de algodon crudo	Grey water-twist or brown cotton yarn.
Hilera en carrisos	Reels of thread or sewing cotton.
Hilera en boletas, blanca	White cotton in balls.
Hilera fina de hilo de dos pelos pā plateros	Silversmiths' wire drawers or plates for drawing wire to the fineness of a hair, of 2 hairs.

Hilo en carrisos	Cotton thread on reels.
Hilo azulado en bolita	Blued white cotton thread in balls.
Hilo ponso	Bright crimson thread.
Hilo amarillo, naranjo	Yellow, orange thread.
Hilo pā emplantillar	Brown shoe thread for sole.
Hilo merlin	Marking thread.
Hilo pitilla, encerado	Waxed "Pitilla" thread.
Hilo cañamazo	Hemp thread.
Hilo acarreto, acaireto	Twine.
Hilo de lana pā carpinteros	Carpenters' lines.
Hilo pā pescar	Fishing line.
Hilo de laton	Wove brass wire.
Hilo de hierro	Wove iron wire.
Hipiometros pā medir alturas con su estuche de cuero	Hypothermometers for measuring heights.
Hisopo	Bottle brush, holy water brush.
Hocenas	Pruning knives.
Hoces pā falhadas	Hedge hooks.
Hoces de picarras	Teethed sickles.
Hoces pā maloja	Sickles for cutting brambles or briars.
Hoces con cabo, pā yerba	Handled sickles, grass sickles.
Hoces pā pesebre con su grampa de espiga	Manger sickles with spike staples.
Hoja, de cuchillo	Blade of any kind, knife blade.
Hoja de parra, loza	Vine-leaf pattern.
Hoja de lata, gruesa y no quebradiza	Tin plate, thick and not battered.
Hoja de cepillos simple	Single plane iron.
Hoja de 3 canales sin vainas	Matchet, 3 furrows, without sheath.
Hoja sin cabo con canal bruñidos	Bright blade without handle.
Hoja de lata calada ó picada	Perforated tin plate.
Hoja de sierra	Web saw.
Hoja de sierra continua	Blade of continuous band saw.
Hoja de plata	Silver foil.
Hoja de cobre	Small copper plate.
Hoja latero	Tinman.
Horca de hierro	Hay pitch-fork.
Horcates de hierro	Iron hames.
Hormas de suncho pā azucar	Sugar funnels, with hoop and nozzle, a canister.
Hormas con alambre y furo	Funnels with hoop iron at point and extra strong wire at mouth.
Hormas con furo de planchuela y suncho doblado en la cabeza	Funnels with hoop iron at point and extra strong wire at mouth.
Horno	Furnace.
Horno de campaña con sus tapas	Camp oven with cover.
Hornillas hierro redondas, cuadradas	Havana stoves, round and square.
Hornillas con sus rejillas aparte	Havana stoves with grates separate.
Hornillas pā fogon	Havana stoves.
Hornillas con 3 pies altos	Braziers' stoves, with 3 long legs.
Horquillas	Hair pins.

Horquillas pa botes	Rowlocks.
Houes polies (F.)	Polished hoes.
Hoyadores ò coas pā café	Coffee diggers.
Hoz	Sickle.
Hueveros, hueveritos	Egg cups.
Hules pā suelo	Oil cloth for floors.
Huacal, Habana	Crate.
Humo negro ò de pez	Lamp black.
Humero	Chimney, smoke funnel.

I

Iman	Loadstone.
Imperial, genero	Imperial, Norfolk imperial shirting
Incienso	Incense.
Incrustados, cuchillos de punta	In-laid tip spear point knives.
Indianas pā enaguas	Indianas regatta prints for under petticoats.
Indianas bandana	Bandano or Swiss cambric prints.
Indianas listadas y encajueladas	Striped or check bandanos for shirtings.
Indianas pā camisas, dibujos grandes	Regatta prints for shirts, large prints.
Indianas menudas y à listas	Regatta prints for shirts, small stripes.
Indianas bandaṇa, nacar y negro	Bandano regatta prints, pearl with black.
Indianas	Regatta cambric or muslin prints.
Indicador de agua, de presion del vapor	Water indicators or indicators of strain pressure.
Ingeniọ, utensilios pā	Articles for sugar estate.
Ingertos de bronce con rosca en la punta	Brass insertion tube with screw at the point.
Instrumentos pā engastador	Chasing tools.
Instrumentos pā medir profundidad de agua	Water gauges.
Instrumentos de talabarteria	Tools, saddlers'.
Instrumentos de jardinero	Gardeners' tools.
Instrumentos pā corta, laminas de cobre	Copper sheet cutting machine.
Instrumentos pā limpiar dientes	Instruments for scaling teeth.
Instrumentos pā sajar	Scarificators.
Irlandas de lino	Irish linen.
Irlandas de algodon	Cotton Irlandas.

J

Jabladeras pā tonelero	Coopers' crosses or groovers.
Jabon almagre, Windsor	Brown Windsor soap.
Jaboneras, de vidrio, de peltre, loza	Soap dishes, glass or pewter, and shaving boxes.
Jacaranda, facas pā carnicero con cabos de	Rose handled butchers' knives.

Jambettes (F.)	Clasp knives.
Jamoneras	Fish kettles, ham boilers.
Jaquimas, jaquimones pā caballo	Halters or head collars.
Jaquimas, jaquimones de cuero con sus cadenas	Halters or head collars with chains
Jaquimon, tornillos pā	Swivel rings.
Jarabe, jarabia, pesos	Syrup, saccharometers.
Jarcia de algodon, cañamo, manila	Coil of cotton, hemp, manilla, rope or cord.
Jarra metal amarillo, pā agua	Yellow metal water jug.
Jarritos	Jugs.
Jarritos pā leche	Cream or milk ewers or jugs.
Jarritos tinta	Ink bottles.
Jarritos lustre	Lustre jugs.
Jarros pico con tapa	Lip jugs with covers.
Jarros delgados y estañados dentro	Copper chocolate pots, tinned.
Jarros grandes	Ewers.
Jarros tanques	Painted jacks, without feet, tall or tankard mugs.
Jarros pā aguamañil	Ewers for wash stand, tin plate.
Jarros malagones, franja color	Tankard mugs, coloured band.
Jarros y palanganas	Ewers and wash basins.
Jarros de lata pintados	Painted tin jacks, jugs, &c.
Jarros de barro pā agua figurando copa	Plain water goblets.
Jarros boca de pato	Ewers with duck shaped mouths.
Jarros de peltre	Pewter jugs.
Jarros pā lavamanos	Toilet jugs.
Jarros de pico pintado	Persian printed lip jugs.
Jarrones	Urns for garden pillars.
Jas en fer (F.)	Iron anvils.
Jaspeado	Marbled, jasper pattern.
Javas de loza	Crates of earthenware.
Javoneras	Soap dishes or boxes.
Jemales, clavos	Jemales nails.
Jibes, gibes ó cedazos	Sieves.
Jicara	Chocolate cup.
Joges pesos de ferro (P.)	Sets iron weights
Jorneleros	Day labourers.
Jorobado, espuelas pico	Bent neck spurs.
Juegos de herrage pā carro, pā coche	Iron work complete, for trucks for coaches.
Juegos pā lavatorios	Sets for wash stands.
Juegos de lavamanos	Toilet sets.
Juegos de mantel	Table cloths.
Juegos completos de cocina	Sets of kitchen fire irons complete.
Juegos de badila, tenazas, tizonero	Sets of shovel, tongs, and poker.
Juegos de parrillas	Sets bars and bearers.
Juegos de ajedrez de marfil	Sets ivory chess men.
Junta de bueyes	Sets or yokes of oxen.
Junteras pā carpintero	Carpenters' jointer planes.

Junquillas,-os	Bead or beading planes.
Junquillos (Buenos Ayres)	Hames.
Junquillos de cadena ò cadenas	Leader hames.
Junquillos de vara ò barra	Shaft or thiller hames.

L

Labores, Indianas de labor	Figuring pattern, Indianas, regatts, prints.
Labrado, dril	Figured drill.
Labrado, cubiertos, con cabo	Fancy tip knives and forks.
Laca	Shellac.
Lacena, alacena, aldabillas pā	Cupboard hooks and eyes.
Lacre colorado en barritas, encarnado	Red sealing wax in sticks.
Ladrillos blancos pā limpiar metales	White bath bricks to clean metals
Ladrillos flojos pā limpiar	Bath bricks.
Ladrillos refractorios ó de fuego	Fire bricks.
Lamina	Sheet metal or plate, leaf, drawing.
Laminado, hierro	Sheet iron or laminated.
Lampas sin palo	Unhandled spades.
Lampas de acero, de cubo	Socket steel spades
Lampas curbas y derechas	Curved and straight spades
Lampas de punta, corrientes	Pointed spades, ordinary quality
Lampas con el fierro en el cabo	Spades with the iron in the handles.
Lamparas giratorias 2 pavilos	Revolving lamps, 2 wicks.
Lamparas pā haciendo	Sugar-house lamps.
Lamparas de pared	Wall lamps.
Lamparas de balanza	Hanging lamps.
Lamparas de movimiento, de colgar	Swing lamps.
Lamparas con bombita y colgador	Lamps with socket and extinguisher.
Lamparas de 1 à 3 luces	1 to 3 light lamps.
Lamparas de corredera	Water-slide lamps.
Lamparas sin corredera	Stiff lamps.
Lamparitas de capuchinas	Small lamps with extinguisher,
Lamparitas giratorias, blancas con apazador y cadenita	White revolving lamps with extinguisher and chain.
Lancetas pā sangrar pā cirujano	Bleeding lances (for surgeons)
Lancetas de 5 cuchillos	Lances of 5 blades.
Lancetas pā caballos	Fleams.
Lanias, lanillas	Muslin de laine.
Lanilla, pā cedazo	Muslin de laine, muslin for sieves.
Lanilla pā bandera Española colorado y amarillo	Bunting for flags, Spanish, red and yellow.
Lanilla, piezas planas	Bunting flat, folded.
Lanilla ò merinos de colores	Coloured merinos.
Lanza	Lance.
Lanza, cuchillos de punta	Spear-point knives.
Lanzaderas y carretillas	Shuttles and reels.
Laña de carpintero	Carpenters' cramp.
Lapiz plomo	Black lead.
Lapiz pā pizarras	Slate pencil.

Lapices buenos pā papel y madera	Good pencils for paper and wood.
Lapices de faltriquera, montados en plata y cilindros de marfil legitimo	Pocket pencils, silver mounted, and barrels of real ivory.
Lapiceros de plata, oro	Silver or gold pencils.
Largavistas	Telescopes.
Largo y longitud	Length.
Largueros	Lengths of any kind.
Latigo de estoque ó espada	Sword whip.
Latigo de martillo	Hammer whip.
Latigo con silbato	Whip with whistle.
Laton, de hierro	Brass, sheet iron.
Lavamanos, lavaderos	Wash stands or toilet sets.
Lavatorios	Wash stands or basins, lavatory.
Lebrillos esmaltados, vidriados	Enamelled pans, glazed pans for washing earthenware and glass.
Lecheras	Milk jugs.
Legitimo, bufaló	Real buffalo.
Lencillos tramados lisos	Plain woven grey domestics.
Lenguetas de picaportes	Small tongues of latches.
Lenguetas pā librero	Bookbinders' knives.
Lentes de aumento, pā miopes	Magnifying glasses or convex for old, concave for young, or short sight.
Lesnas pā zapatero, pā talabartero	Shoemakers' awls, saddlers' awls.
Lesnas pā tacon	Heel awls.
Lesnas pā encuadernador, encavernador	Bookbinders' awls.
Lesnas pā palmillas	Pegging awls.
Lesnas sin ò con cabos	Handled or unhandled awls.
Lesnas sables	Sword-shape awls.
Lesnas curbas, lingua de vibora	Sewing viper-tongue bent awls.
Letreso	The lettering of a sign, &c.
Levita	Frock coat, &c.
Lebrito de amigo, de memoria	Album, pocket book.
Libro de dibujos	Book of drawings, pattern book.
Licor	Dram glass.
Licorera con botellas	Liquor frame with bottles.
Lienzas ordinarias pā medir	Measuring tapes.
Lienzas ò medidas de cinta	Measure tapes.
Lienzas con caja de suela	Measure tapes with leather case.
Ligadura	Bandage.
Lija de vidrio con lienzo	Glass cloth.
Lija esmeril de trapo	Emery cloth.
Limas almendrillo, atonendrillo ½ redondas	Pit saw files, taper pit or mill saw files, or almond-shaped or tumbler
Limas com agranzo atravesado (P.)	Diagonal cut or grain files.
Limas Pottance, Globe, Brittain	Pottance, Globe, Brittain files.
Limas planas, medias, suaves	Flat half-smooth, second-cut files.
Limas grano fino, gordo	Fine cut, rough cut, or grain files.
Limas tablas pā serrote de una raya	Single cut files, cross-cut saw files.

Limas rabo de raton	Rat-tail files.
Limas punta aguda	Sharp-point files.
Limas chatas picadura entre fina	Flat files, middle fine cut for blacksmiths.
Limas musas tablas de un corte y canto redondo	Flat smooth files of one cut and round edge.
Limas ½ caña triangulares	Half-round, triangular files.
Limas pica gruesa	Rough-cut or grain files.
Limas pā marmolistas	Files for statuary.
Limas un canto liso	Files with one smooth edge.
Limas bastardas	Bastard files.
Limadura de bronce, de hierro	Brass, iron filings.
Limatones	Pit-saw files.
Limeria	Files.
Limpia dedos	Finger glasses.
Limpia pies bronceados	Bronzed foot scrapers.
Lines de algodon	Cotton lines.
Lingotes de hierro fundido de cabeza pā parrillas	Cast-iron furnace bars with head.
Lingotes de Gartsherrie	Gartsherrie pig-iron.
Lino liso blanco y linon liso blanco	Plain white leno, plain white book muslin.
Lino de obispo	Bishop's lawn.
Linoes bordados	Embroidered lenos.
Linternas hoja de lata, vidrio de cacho	Tin lanterns, horn leaf.
Linternas pā sereno	Watchman's lanterns.
Linternas mudas	Dark lanterns.
Linternas pā cuartos de niños con lampara pā mover arriba y abajo y tetera ò jarrito pā papilla	Nursery lamps.
Lios de 6 arrobas, barras mineros cortadas en	Ties of 6 arrobas, (miners' bars, cut in.)
Lirones ò gatos	Lifting jacks.
Liso	Plain or smooth.
Listas, dril à listas	Striped drill.
Listado de hilo, de algodon	Striped linen or cotton drill or check.
Listitas tinto morado	Claret - coloured, purple, small stripes, listitas.
Listo	Ready.
Liston de pana	Velvet ribbon.
Liston de pana negra labrada	Black embroidered cotton velvet ribbon or tapes.
Listones de raso	Satin stripes.
Listones ó molduras	Beading planes.
Litargirio ó sea secante en polvo	Litharge or dryer, oxide of lead in powder.
Llamadores de metal	Brass knockers.
Llantas de carreta	Waggon wheel tyres.
Llaves pā cerraduras	Keys for locks.

Llaves pā barriles, pipas, &c.	Cocks for barrels, pipes, &c.
Llaves pā embotellar	Bottling cocks.
Llaves con pico, largo, corto, enterizo	Cocks with long, short, entire, nose or spout.
Llaves de vapor con palanca	Steam cocks with levers.
Llaves hierro de concesion	Iron gas main cocks.
Llaves metal de continuacion, pā gas	Continuation brass cocks for gas pipes.
Llaves de continuacion pā gas, &c.	Stop cocks.
Llaves de hierro pā destornillar	Iron wrenches for unscrewing, turnscrews.
Llaves pā desarmar camas	Keys to take down and fit up bedsteads.
Llaves pā prueba de vapor	Steam-proof cocks.
Llaves indicadores de agua y tubos de vidrio	Water indicators, cocks and tubes of glass.
Llaves de presion	Pression or spring cocks.
Llaves de derrame pā desagué	Bib cocks.
Llaves de quita y pon	Cocks for pipes with loose key.
Llaves de fusil	Cocks of gun.
Llaves de metal con platillos pā tanques	Brass cocks with flange for tanks.
Llaves de alimentor	Feeding cocks.
Llaves pā mamparas	Brass knob and spindle for fire screens.
Llaves pā manguera	Rotatory stop cocks, with unions on one end.
Llaves de prueba de agua y tubos	Waterproof cocks and tubes.
Llaves pā botar el agua y tubo	Cocks for throwing the water, and tube.
Llaves de laton, de metal, de bronce, de 2 platillos	Brass cocks for country houses or estates, 2 flanges.
Llaves pā placeres	Brass cocks with 2 flanges.
Llaves de prueba verticales con palanca y tapon	Vertical proof cocks, with key and plug.
Llaves pā dar cuerda à reloj	Watch keys.
Llaves caneria de gas, piperia, tuberia de agua	Cocks for gas or water piping or tubing.
Llaveros de acero	Steel key rings.
Locetas, lozetas	Paving tiles.
Lona de hilo pā vela, gante	Sacking or sail cloth.
Loza pintada	Painted earthenware.
Loza fina	Printed earthenware.
Loza, tibores, servicios	Bidet pans.
Loza, tazas pā café	Tea cups.
Loza ½ china	China.
Loza, tazas	Cups and saucers or teas.
Lozas pā bidet, ò bidel	Bidet pans.
Lozas, losas	Flagstones of earthenware.
Lozetas ò locetas	Paving tiles.
Luciferas de cera	Lucifer matches, wax matches or vestas.

Lunas pã espejos	Glass plates for mirrors.
Lunas pã lamparas	Domes, glass globes for lamps.
Lustrada, loza	Lustre earthenware.
Lustre, jarros de	Lustre jugs.
Lustroso	Bright, shining.
Luz, luces	Light, inside diameter of hole or bore.

M

Macanas, hierro acerado	Steeled iron coffee diggers.
Maceta de mano	Hand mallet.
Machados	Tomahawks or hand hatchets.
Machetes con espiga	Matchets with spike or tang.
Machetes pã chapear curbos, cabo de tarro, de chapeo	Horn handled bent matchets.
Machetes rayados, cabo de cuerno	Horn handled ribbed matchets.
Machetes de canales, con rete	Matchets with furrow.
Machetes desmochados	Cut point matchets.
Machetes momposinos	Mompos matchets, white bone handled.
Machetes pã cocina	Kitchen cleavers.
Macheticos de monte	Hunting knives.
Machihembradas, macho y hembras sin manijas	Grooving planes without handles.
Machos pã herrero	Pane hammers.
Machos, visagras con	Hook and eye hinges.
Madapolames, madapollames, madapolanes	Madapolams, shirtings.
Madejas, hilo en	Linen thread in hanks or skeins.
Madejitas pã carpintero	Carpenter's lines.
Maderaje	Wood work.
Madres pã lingotes, parrillas	Bearers for furnace bars and bearers
Magnesia calcinada	Calcined magnesia.
Mailles, chaines divisèes par (F.)	Connecting links or shackles, chains divided by.
Majadero, morteros con	Pestle, mortars with.
Majado	Bruised or pounded.
Majorcas de cacao, cuchillos cabo de cubo pã tirar	Knives to cut ears of cocoa.
Malagones	Tall mugs.
Maletas	Portmanteaus, carpet bags.
Maleticas	Small travelling valises.
Malettes (F.)	Tinned boxes, japanned oak.
Mallas, tela alambre laton de 30	Meshes, brass wove wire, 30 meshes to the inch.
Mamparas	Door screens, or green baize doors, glass doors or sashes.
Mana en lagrimas, canutillo, suerte,	Manna in drops, stick, natural state.
Manches de corne (F.)	Horn handles.
Machettes oú machetes (F.)	Matchets.
Mancillas	Cranks.

Mancuernillas, gemelos	Sleeve buttons, pairs.
Mandarrias de 2 bocas	Two-faced stone hammers,
Mandarrias boca de un lado y redondas por otro	Stone hammers, mouth on one side and round on other.
Mandarrias de boca y piña	Stone hammers, with flat and sharp or pointed end.
Mandarrias boca redonda	Stone hammers, with round mouth.
Mandarrias de hierro pă calafates	Iron caulking hammers.
Mandiles	Saddle cloths.
Mangos de quita y pon	Lift-off handles.
Mangos pă plumas	Penholders.
Mangos pă quitrin	Gig handles.
Mangueras, tubos pă	Hose tubes.
Manicomios	Manometer for small steam engines.
Maniguetas pă sierra de aire	Handles, pit saw boxes and tillers complete.
Manijas ó manejas pă baul, &c.	Handles for trunks, &c.
Manillitas ò chapitas pă ataudes	Plated coffin handles.
Manillos	Handcuffs.
Manipuladores	Manipulators for telegraph.
Mano de papel	Quire of paper.
Manta dril blanca doble, muy tupida	Double white drill manta, very stout manta.
Manta doble rasa, cruda, manta dril crudo	Manta, stout grey domestics, unbleached drill.
Manta de lana	A blanket, woollen.
Manteles, juegos de	Sets table cloths.
Mantillas pă caballo	Saddle cloths.
Mantequilleras, mantequillas	Butter tubs or coolers.
Manuables, surtido de martillos	Assortment of hand hammers.
Manubrios	Crank handles of fly wheels or the handles of the cranks.
Maque ó maqueado, papel	Papier maché.
Maquina de (pă) moler caña de azucar	Horizontal sugar mills.
Maquina pă hilar algodon	Cotton spinning machine.
Maquina de café	Coffee machine.
Maquina pă cardar	Carding machine.
Maquina de trillar	Threshing machine.
Maquina pă eventar	Winnowing.
Maquina de descascarar cañamo	Hemp breaking machine.
Maquina pă cortar yerba	Grass cutting machine.
Maquina pă cortar paja	Chaff cutting machine.
Maquina corte, estampa	Cutting, stamping machine.
Maquina neumatica	Air pump.
Maquina pă cortar plumas de ganso	Machine for cutting goose quills.
Maquina pă afilar cuchillos	Patent knife sharpener.
Maquina pă levantar pesos	Windlass.
Maquina pă agujerear	Punching machine.
Maquina pă cortar y dividir el cuero pă talabartero	Cutting and splitting machine for saddlers.

68

Maquina pā estirar y partir el cuero	Straining and splitting machine.
Maquina pā separar los tamaños del grano de café	Coffee sizing machine.
Maquina de alambrar	Wiring machine.
Maquina cortadora circular	Circle cutter.
Maquina seguradora de fondas	Bottom closer.
Maquina dobleadora de codo	Angle bender,
Maquina machihembradora	Grooving machine.
Maquina pā hacer tapa de pimientera	Machine for making pepper box heads.
Maquina pā hacer pico de tetera	Teapot neck or spout tool.
Maquina pā hacer embudo	Funnel stake.
Maquina pā hacer medias lunas	Half-moon stake.
Maquina pā hacer cabezas redondas	Round head stake.
Maquina pā hacer apagadores	Extinguisher stake.
Maquina dobleadora, pā doblar	Folder.
Maquinitas pā rizar ropa	Goffering machine.
Maquinitas pa fechar los papelitos	Machine for dating tickets.
Marcas pā fuego	Branding irons.
Marcas	Labels on goods, also trade mark.
Marcadores pā madera	Timber scribes.
Marcos de metal, de peso pā balanza	Frames, brass cup weights.
Marcos pā estirar	Drawing frames.
Marcos con puertas	Furnace door frames.
Marcos, argollas pā	Rings with screw for picture frames.
Marcos con vidrio	Glazed frames with mats.
Marfil	Ivory.
Marfiles	Ivory combs.
Marmas ò marmitas de lata	Camp kettles.
Marmites fonte emaillées (F.)	Cast enamelled round pots.
Marquesas hierro	Bedsteads.
Marraño, sillas cuero de	Hogskin saddles.
Marrones ò cubos de hierro	Blacksmiths' hammers, sledge hammers.
Marroqui, maroquin, tafilete	Morocco.
Marta oscura, pinceles de 2 puntas	Brushes of 2 points of dark sable.
Marteaux à calfat (F.)	Caulking mallets.
Martillos pā herrero	Blacksmiths' hammers.
Martillos pā calzado claveteados	Shoe hammers pinned.
Martillos de tapicero	Upholsterers' hammers.
Martillos de uña, oreja pua, sin cabo	Unhandled claw hammers, Kent hammers.
Martillos de tenaza	Oval-headed axe.
Martillos de ojo	Eye hammers.
Martillos pā estaquillar	Pegging hammers.
Martillos de cantero	Stone hammers.
Martillo, hierro à	Wrought-iron.
Martinete de vapor con martillo	Steam hammer.
Martingalas	Martingales.
Marvetes	Labels.

Masa, masilla, vejiga de	Bladder of putty.
Maseteros pā flores	Flower stands.
Mason, cirage en boite de fer blanc	Paste of blacking, in tin boxes.
Masos,-zos	Sledge hammers.
Masos pa hacer balastro	Mallets or hammers for making road metal.
Matizados de amarillo pañuelos de bandera encarnada	Red Bandana handkerchiefs with yellow design.
Matizado	Different tinted.
Matriz	Worm of a screw.
Maza chica, guijos pā	Small rollers, shafts for.
Mazilla, masilla	Putty.
Mazisos, picos pā sangear canteros	Solid iron picks for quarries.
Mazos de fleje	Bundles of hoop iron, less than atado.
Mazos de herrero	Sledge or smith's hammers.
Mazos de carreta	Naves of waggon wheels.
Mazos pā moler metales	Stampers.
Mazos, guijos pā	Shafts and centres for small rollers.
Mecedores, sillones	Rocking chairs.
Mechas	Centre bits.
Mechas pā berbiquies, en cada docena un atornillador y un abillanador	Brace bits, in each dozen a screw driver and a countersink or almond-shaped bit.
Mechas pā barrenas	Safety fuze.
Mechas de algodon	Cotton wicks.
Mechas solares	Solar cottons or wicks.
Mechas de cera	Wax matches, vestas.
Meches de Vilbrequin à la cuilliére	Brace bits, spoon shape.
Mecheros metal amarillo	Brass lamp burners.
Mecheros pā sacar candela	Tinder boxes with flint and steel.
Mechoneros	Tinder boxes with flint and steel.
Medias blancas de algodon muy finas pā señoras	Very fine ladies white cotton stocking, small foot, without seam.
Medias de cordon algodon	Ribbed hose, cotton.
Medias de lana pā hombres lisas	Men's worsted hose, plain.
Medias medias de algodon	Cotton socks.
Medias lunas con sus muelles y chapas pā cajones de escritorio, de comoda	Half moons, with their springs and plates, for escritoire drawers.
Media china	China.
Media caña, limas '	Half-round files.
Medios puntos de metal pā carpeta	Brass quadrants and catches for desks.
Medidas de boz pā carpinteros	Carpenters' 3 feet box rules.
Medidas redondas de alambre	Round wire gauges.
Medidas pā medir hierro	Rule with slide for measuring iron.
Medidas pā medir à 100lbs., agua	Brass circular steam gauge up to 100 lbs., water gauge.
Medidas de agrimensores	Land surveyor's measures.
Medidas de cinta ò lienzas	Measure tapes.

Medidor alambre	Wire gauge.
Melado, loza	Dipped, earthenware.
Melchor, palmatorias de	German silver chamber candlesticks
Ménudos y listas, dibujos Indianas	Regatta prints, small and striped pattern.
Mercado de hierro	Iron market.
Mercurio dulce	Calomel.
Merino ó cobourg	Merino or cobourg.
Merino ó lanillas de colores	Coloured merinos in imitation of the French.
Merlines, pā nopal	Muslins, merlines, book muslins.
Merma	A going in, in weight or bulk.
Mesa pā adorno de una sala	Drawing room table.
Mesa de hesillo, de juego	Card table.
Mesa de ajedrez	Chess table.
Mesa giratoria	Revolving platform, (rail.)
Mesitás de labor	Work tables.
Mesitas de papier maché	Small papier mache tables.
Metal agrio, dulce	Brass, any metal, unannealed, annealed.
Metal blanco ó plata alemana	White metal or German silver.
Metal campañil	Bell metal.
Mezclilla pā pantalones	Mixtures for trousers.
Millo, bruzas de raiz de millo	Dandy brushes, made of the roots of millet or pannic grass.
Mimbre	Wicker.
Minoria de flete	The smallness of the freight.
Minio, miñon, minium pā hacer juntos de tubos	Minnum or red lead for joining pipes.
Mitad, azadas mitad bruñidas	Half-polished hoes.
Mobile, loza	Mobile.
Modico, hierro del	Cheapest iron.
Moinhos pā café (P.)	Coffee mills.
Moldes pā velas	Candle moulds.
Moldes pā azucar	Sugar funnels or moulds.
Moldes pā hacer balas	Bullet moulds.
Molduras con rebajador pā mamparas de vidrio con hierros	Sash planes with irons.
Molduras ò listones	Beading planes.
Molduras pā carpinteros	Carpenters' Grecian moulding planes.
Molduras quiales	Quirk moulding planes.
Molinete, molinito	Crane for lifting, windlass.
Molinos pā maiz, café, &c.	Mills for Indian corn, coffee.
Molinos pā pintura	Colour mills.
Molinos pā café pā poner en horcon	Post iron coffee mills.
Molinos de columna pā clavar en poste	Post iron coffee mills.
Molinos con cajon de hierro y tubo de laton	Mill with iron box and brass hopper.
Molinos con embudo	Mill with funnel.

Molinos pā engranage	Mill for grain.
Molinos pā moler cebada, avena, guisantes	Mill for crushing barley, oats, and peas.
Molinos con armadura de hierro pā moler maiz	Mill for crushing Indian corn, with iron fittings.
Molinos pā triturar corteza de roble	Mill for grinding oak bark.
Mollejones finos	Fine grinding stones.
Montados de metal	Brass mounts.
Montones charolados pā guarda barra de coches	Japanned basils for splash boards of coaches.
Monturas pā señoras (Guay.)	Ladies' saddles.
Moqueta	Cloth for binding.
Morado lirio	Purple, lily purple.
Morcillas ó chorizos, maquina pā hacer	Black pudding and pork sausage, machine for making.
Mordazas ò eclises hierro dulce	Wrought-iron fish bars or plates.
Mordazas	Silversmiths' nippers.
Morrales	Valises, game bags.
Morriones	Military caps or shakoes.
Mors acier avec filets acier (F.)	Steel bits with steel snaffles or curbs
Morteros de pasta Inglesa, morteros pā farmacia	Apothecaries' mortars, composition.
Morteros con sus manos	Mortars and pestles.
Mortuarios pā ataudes, juegos de	Sets of coffin furniture.
Mosquiteros	Mosquito curtains.
Mostacillas	Small beads, assorted, red, white, blue, &c.
Mostruario de quincalleria	Set of musters or patterns, hardware.
Mostruario completo de papel pā cartas, sobres y plumas	Showcase of letter paper, envelopes and steel pens.
Motones charolados, extra grandes	Extra large japanned basils or roans
Motones pā tapafondos de sillas	Tanned basils or roans to cover saddles.
Motones extra grandes pā guarda-barra de coches	Japanned basils for splash boards of coaches.
Motones ó mutones blancos	White basils or roans.
Motones lisos color de cascara	Tanned basils or roans, shell colour
Motones hierro con roldanas de metal	Iron pulleys with brass wheels.
Motones de pozo con ganchos	Well blocks and hooks.
Motones pā buques con ganchos	Ship blocks and hooks.
Motones hierro ruedas de metal	Iron pulley blocks, brass wheels.
Motones hierro pā aparejos de pozo	Iron pulleys for well gear.
Mouchettes (F.)	Reed planes.
Muebles	House furniture.
Muefles	Muffles.
Mueles pā cortar hierro	Chisels for cutting iron.
Muelle	Spring, also a wharf.
Muelle real	Mainspring, as of gun lock
Muelle de reloj	Watch spring.

Muelle hechura de reloj	Watch-shape spring.
Muesca	Mortice.
Muestra	Muster, pattern, dial of a watch.
Municion pã cazar aves grandes y pequeños	Shot for large and small birds.
Municion pã venado	Shot for deer or stags.
Municioneras	Shot pouches or belts.
Muñecos tinteros	Inkstands in the form of little figures.
Muñon de guijo	Lug or ear of coffee mill shaft.
Musarola	Ornament for harness.
Muselinas	Muslins.
Muselinas estampadas de colores	Printed or coloured muslins.

N

Nabajas ó navajas cortaplumas finas	Fine penknives.
Nabajas cuchillos de gonce que cierran	Knives with spring at back to shut.
Nacar fino, grana	Scarlet, fine red
Nacar paño	Scarlet cloth.
Nacar	Pearl shell.
Naguas, enaguas	Petticoats.
Narizeras	Iron nose rings.
Natural, color	Self colour, natural.
Navajas de afeitar ó pã barba	Razors.
Navajas, cachas de mucha fantasia	Knives, very fancy handles.
Navajas pã jardines, jardinero	Gardeners' pruning knives.
Navajas pã gallo	Cock spurs.
Navajas pã marinero	Sailors' knives.
Navajas con asentador	Razors with strop.
Navajas en estuche de baul	Razors in trunk shape case.
Navalhas de gancho (P.)	Pocket pruning knives.
Necesarios pã viage	Canteens.
Neceseres de cuero con avios pã hombres	Men's leather dressing case furnished.
Negro humo	Lamp black.
Neptunas	Neptune coal scoops.
Nivel de aire embutido en caja pã la nivelacion con reglas en las obras delicadas	Air levels inlet into a case for exact leveling in nice work.
Nivel de agua, de espiritu	Water level, spirit level.
Niveladores que no sean falsos	Levels, true.
Nomina	List.
Nuez y sobre nuez	Nut of main spring of gun lock.
Nuez de plomado	Wooden nut, reel of plummets,
Nuez moscada	Nutmeg.
Nudos de hierro	Iron snipes.
Nudos goznes	Snipes.

O

Objectivo y su camara	Lens and camera.
Obleas	Wafers.

ͻ	Skew.
϶ caldero	Braziers' work.
ɖo	Octagon.
narillo	Yellow ochre.
jetes, ojetillas, blancos, pá tos	White eyelets for shoes.
perdiz	Bird's eye lenses
almendra	Almond eye.
Iolan, liso	Plain muslin.
	Camp ovens, round bellied pots.
randes con pies	Large round pots with legs.
e hierro con porcelana	Enamelled round bellied pots.
e rabo y asa	Long and bow-handled pots.
os asas esmaltados por dentro	Enamelled inside and bow-handled round bellied pots.
hierro con porcelana, loza, lo	Enamelled iron pots.
ɔá colero	Glue pots.
hierro estañadas con orejas acer chocolate	Tined iron chocolate pots with bow handles.
ios	Workmen.
	Opium.
s de seaux (F.)	Kettle ears or lugs.
	Ear or handle.
ızul y verde, fuentes, platos	Blue and green edge dishes.
es ò orinallos borde chato ó ndo	Flat or round rim chambers.
es, templo y marruecos	Chambers, Temple and Morocco
es chatos	Bed pans,
as blancas, Victoria	Victoria lawns.
hilaza cruda	Ball brown thread.
res pá café	Coffee diggers.

P

ferro (P)	Iron shovel.
cisco (P)	Dust shovel.
ado	Blued.
hilo de coser vela	Bundles, packages, sail thread.
pá señora	Ladies' billiard cues.
estañadas	Tinned sugar pans.
hierro colado, borde rasgado	Cast iron, sugar pans sloping flange
hierro colado, borde virado	Cast iron sugar pans, turned over rims.
ó peroles	Preserving pans.
de carron probadas	Carron proved sugar pans.
de paños	Wrought iron sugar pans.
esfericas	Spherical pans.
de vapor	Steam boilers.
figura ahuevada	Egg-shaped sugar pans.
figura batea	Trough-shaped sugar pans.
pá fregar	Pans for cleaning, sponging.

Pailitas	Preserving pans.
Pailitas	Small sugar pans.
Pailitas pā cocinar, pā cocina	Kitchen pans, cooking pans.
Pailitas de cobre pā preservas	Copper preserving pans.
Paja, color	Straw colour
Palas pā tierra	Gravel shovels.
Palas pā zanjear	Grafting tools.
Palas ¼ luna	Grafting tools or half-moon shovels
Palas pā jardin	Garden spades.
Palas ahuecadas	Scooped out coal shovels.
Palas de mano, pā basura	Dust or dung shovels or pans.
Palas pā cavar	Digging shovels.
Palas de ribete	Shovels with seam or border.
Palas pā trabajadores	Labourers' shovels.
Palas de cuchara pā azucar	Spoon-shape sugar shovels.
Palas pā eventar	Winnowing, corn shovels.
Palas pā palear, apalear	Shovelling shovels with socket.
Palas pā puntear, puntar	Spades with ring socket.
Palas pā lidiar taguas	Demerara trenching shovels or open socket spades.
Palas punta redonda, mitad con mango muletilla, mitad agujereado	Shovels, half crutch, half eye, tree handle.
Palas con mango de muleta, de ojo	Shovels, crutch, eye tree handle.
Palas de maniguetas	Handled shovels.
Palas de nariz redonda	Round nose shovels.
Palas de cuchara	The bowls of spoons.
Palas de fornalla	Furnace shovels.
Palas plates, bien aceradas, courbes	Flat and bent shovels well steeled.
Palas angostas	Spades.
Palas ò cucharones pā recoger dinero	Shovels to take up money with.
Paladeo, loza	Toy (earthenware)
Palanca, llaves con	Cocks with lever.
Palanca y pilon, romanos con	Steelyards with lever and ball
Palanca de hierro	Iron crow bar.
Palanca de triple cambiavias	Lever for triple switches.
Palangana y jarro	Wash basin and ewer.
Palangana borde virado	Round rim wash basin.
Palanganeros habilitadas	Fitted-up portable washstands.
Palanquetas pā trabajos de jimnasia	Dumb-bells.
Palanquinatas hierro fundido	Cast iron bowls, preserving pans.
Palaustres pā albañil	Masons' trowels.
Paletas	Painters' knives.
Palitas con agujeros	Small shovels with holes inside.
Palitas de mano charoladas	Japanned hand shovels for fire.
Palitas pā plumas de acero	Steel pen holders.
Palma, aceite de	Palm oil.
Palmatorias	Chamber candlesticks.
Palmatorias con bombilla giratoria y cadenita	Chamber candlesticks, with revolving socket and chain.
Palo mora	Fustic,

Palo Brasil	Logwood or Brasil wood.
Pana de palo á cuadros	Cotton velvet, check pattern.
Panas negras labradas	Black figured stuffs.
Panas	Tinned basins.
Panadera	Bread basket.
Panellas ou caçarollas (P.)	Stewpans, round iron pots.
Paniers à fruits (F.)	Bread or fruit baskets.
Pantallas de chimenca con pedestal	Fire screens with foot.
Pantallas de papel (P.)	Paper shades for lamps.
Pantometras, reglas	Pantometer rules.
Panturrias con macho y hembra	Hook and eye hinges.
Panurges vernies et plaquées argent (F.)	Japanned and plated loops for harness.
Pañalones, merino	Shawls, merino.
Paño	Cloth, sheet of metal, &c.
Paño ancho, negro, azul, gris, &c.	Wide cloth, black, blue, grey, &c.
Paño de mano	Towel.
Paño de cobre	Copper sheet.
Pañuelos en gasa ó muselina y coquillo estampado	Handkerchiefs, muslin and printed coquillo, or jaconet and cambric.
Pañuelos corbata	Neckerchiefs.
Pañuelos de bandana encarnados ó nacar, matizados de amarillo y verde	Red bandana handkerchiefs, with yellow and green designs.
Pañuelos con guardas y dibujos amarillos	Bandana handkerchiefs, yellow borders and designs.
Pañuelos de hilo	Linen handkerchiefs.
Pañuelos de fondo blanco	White ground handkerchiefs.
Pañuelos de lana	Worsted shawls.
Pañuelos de marca mayor, labor nacar y azul	Coloured lappet shawls, pink and blue.
Pañuelos de burato liso	Plain Burato crape shawls.
Pañuelos de seda de la India	India silk handkerchiefs.
Pañuelos de seda blanca	White silk handkerchiefs.
Pañuelos de seda cruda	Printed corah handkerchiefs.
Pañuelones de gros	Worsted shawls.
Pañuelones de burato lisos con fleco	Plain crape Burato shawls with fringe.
Papel de genero blanco	White linen paper.
Papel de cartas rayado, pā cartas, billetes	Ruled letter paper, letter paper.
Papel de marca pā dibujo	Paper suitable for drawing.
Papel pā dibujar, de dibujo	Drawing paper.
Papel de trazar	Tracing paper.
Papel de copiar	Copying paper.
Papel dioptrico, azulado pā calcar	Dioptric blued tracing paper.
Papel secante	Blotting paper.
Papel fino de gusto con guardias, juego de	Set of fine tasty paper with border, for house.
Papel de arrimo	Hanging paper.

Papel basto de estraza	Brown paper.
Papel de forro	Packing, sheathing paper.
Papel ò papelon de empaquetar	Strong packing paper.
Papel continuo frances ò ingles forrado en lienzo	Continuous French or English paper, lined with linen.
Papel de trapo esmeril	Emery cloth.
Papel de esmeril	Emery paper
Papel de lija de trapo, trapo de lija	Glass cloth.
Papel de lija	Glass paper.
Papel maseado	Papier mache.
Papilitos,-as	Tickets, labels.
Papilitos de pergamio pā poner marcas	Parchment labels for marking.
Papilla ó rejilla pā asiento de sillas	Cane wove bottoms of chairs.
Paquetes de alfileres de 12 peines	Packets of pins, 12 rows.
Paquetitos, tachuela cortada estañada	Small packets cut tinned tacks
Paraceniza	Fender.
Paradas perches	Parchment receivers or stops.
Paragua, amazon de ballena	Umbrella, whalebone frame.
Paraguero	Umbrella stand.
Pararayos	Lightning conductor.
Parrillas, figura de sable, de cuchillo, vitrubio	Sword, knife shape, bars and bearers
Parrillas hierro colado pā madres	Cast iron bars and bearers
Parrillas pā cocina con loza de patente	Gridirons, patent enamelled
Parrillas ordinarias, girantes	Common revolving gridirons.
Parrillas pā calentar tostado	Footmen to fix on fenders for toasting.
Partenueces	Nutcrackers.
Pasa por todo	Compass or key-hole saw.
Pasas, cedazos pā	Sieves for raisins.
Pasas cardas	Wool cards.
Pasadores de uña, pā embutir	Flush bolts.
Pasadores rectos	Straight bolts.
Pasadores de rabo largo, chapa angosta, perilla metal	Long-tail bolts, narrow plate and brass knob.
Pasadores chatos con rabo y perilla	Flat tail bolts with knob.
Pasadores de resorte, muelle	Spring bolts.
Pasadores orientales, con rabo	Monkey-tail bolts, India bolts.
Pasadores con hembra	Bolts with eyes.
Pasadores cuadrados á la francesa	Square French bolts.
Pasadores de laton, metal, pā vidriera	Barrel sash fasteners.
Pasadores de plata (Lima)	Silver;tips.
Pasadores pā estriberas	Stirrup slides.
Pasamano de metal pā balcones	Brass hand rail for balconies.
Pasaportes	Spring bolts or latches.
Paseadores pā perros	Dog swivels.

Passe travers, martillos pā herrero	Cross pane hammers.
Pasteleras con pie	Pie dishes.
Pavas de laton	Brass tea kettles.
Pavas cafeteras, asa fija sin cilindro	Tea kettles, fixed lacquered handle, not cylinder.
Pavilo	Wick of candle or lamp.
Pavon azul ò pavonado	Blued.
Peaux de moutons vernis (F.)	Basils or roans.
Pecho de angel, fleco	Angel breast fringe.
Pedazos de cobre chato	Pieces flat brass, copper.
Pedernal azul, Turqui	Flown blue, Turkey blue.
Pedernal, loza de	Stone ware.
Pediluvio, juego de	Foot bath set.
Pedrero	Swivel gun.
Peines pā tocador	Dressing combs.
Peines escarpidores de goma	India rubber dressing combs.
Peines espesas	Fine tooth combs.
Peines marfil	Ivory combs.
Peines de bolsillo	Pocket combs.
Peines asta, carei, tortulla	Horn, tortoise, turtle shell combs.
Peines de imitacion tortuga	Imitation tortoise shell combs.
Peines pā pintura	Steel painting combs or grainers' tools.
Peinillas	Small tooth combs.
Peinillas de cuerno negro	Black horn dress combs.
Peinillas caguamo, imitacion carei, arqueadas	Stained dressing comb, roach back.
Peldaños pā cama	Bed steps.
Pelles (F.)	Shovels, spades.
Pelo, alambre hierro cobrizado de pelo	Silk-covered hair wire for artificial flowers.
Pelotas pā niños	Playing balls for children.
Peltre	Britannia metal, pewter.
Pendientes ó zarcillos	Ear rings.
Pentures á pattes (F.)	Hook and eye hinges with plate.
Pentures et gonds en fer (F.)	Hook and eye hinges with jagged spike.
Peña, piña	Sharp end of stone hammer.
Peon ò eje vertical	Vertical axle.
Perāmbuladores mimbre, sencillos	Light basket work perambulators.
Percalas de algodon	Nine-eight cotton percolas or prints.
Percalas listadas y á cuadros	Fancy check and stripe muslins.
Percalas ojo de perdiz	Bird's eye lenos.
Perchas pā ropa	Hat and coat hooks.
Perdigoneras con sus correas	Shot belts with leathers.
Perillas, de laton, de palo	Brass, wood knobs.
Perrillos, machetes	One-furrow, long narrow matchets with dog stamped on them.
Perlas imitacion nacar	Pearl imitation beads.
Perillas ó remates de laton, cristal blanco, madera negra, porcelana blanca	Knobs, brass, white or clear crystal, ebony, porcelain.

Perillas, parrillas	Gridirons.
Pernos de carreta	Waggon, linch, or cotter pins.
Peroles hierro batido	Wrought-iron preserving pans, salt and sugar pans.
Peroles de cobre estañado	Tinned copper pots for distilling.
Peroles perolitas, medias	Small, half preserve pans.
Peroles pā trapiche con cinchas y orejas	Sugar pans with belly bands and lugs or ears.
Pertigos	Cart poles
Pertinencias, molinos con sus	Mills complete.
Pesa siropes, guarapos, jarabes,-ia	Saccharometer.
Pesa licor, instrumento pā pesar licores	Hydrometer.
Pesas pā oro	Gold scales.
Pesas de metal españolas en mar-, quitos de una libra	Brass Spanish weights in sets of 1-lb. downwards.
Pesas de laton, de hierro	Brass, iron, weights.
Pesas,-os, pā encajar	Cup weights.
Pesas,-os, de resorte	Spring balances.
Pescaderas con coladores y tapas	Fish kettles or dishes with strainers and covers.
Pescantes pā mosquitero	Scroll for mosquito curtains.
Peseantes pā muelles	Cranes for weighing, for quays, wharfs.
Pesebre, hoces pā	Manger, stable, sickles.
Pestillos, langueta	Link, latches ; tongue link.
Pez rubia	Red, amber resin.
Pica gruesa, limas tablas	Rough-cut flat files.
Picados, picoteados, clavos pā llantas	Jagged tyre nails.
Picaportes de muletilla con chapa de asiento	Crutch latches with their plate.
Picaportes con 2 bolas	Latches with 2 knobs.
Picaportes de bolitas con lenguetas y platillos	Latches with small knobs, tongues and plates.
Picaportes pā vidriera de lenguetas con argolla	Cupboard turns, window catches, sash fasteners, with tongues and ring.
Picaportes con pomo y langueta	Sash fasteners, cupboard turns.
Picaportes pā ventanas	Latches for windows.
Picaportes pā noche	Night latches.
Picaportes de hierro	Solid end iron tower bolts.
Pico	Lip, (earthenware) ; neck of sput.
Pico, de 4 hasta 3 y pico	From 4 to 3 and a fraction.
Picos, ratoneras pā ratones, ratas, zorros, prenzas con picos	Traps for mice, rats, foxes, the catch with teeth.
Picos, llaves con picos cortos, largos	Cocks with long, short spout.
Picos, pā arado	Ploughshares or plough points.
Picos con lampa pā sanjear canteros	Miners' picks with flat or spade end.
Pie de amigo con su abrazadera y flor, ó planchuela de sosten	Sign or lamp bracket.
Pie de gato	Trigger of a gun.

Pie de rey	Folding box rule.
Pie de cabra	Boot jack.
Piedras pā zapateros, enteras	Shoemakers' lapstones.
Piedras de agujar	Whetstones.
Piedras pā afilar y asentar, nabajas de barba	Razor hones with strop.
Piedras azulosas, azules	Carpenters' blue stones.
Piedras de Hindostan	Green oilstones.
Piedras sueltas con abrazadera y argollita pā sacar chispa	Loose agate flint with clasp and ring for attaching them, for striking fire.
Piedras de chispa pā fusil, color caramela	Straw-coloured gun flints.
Piedras de Turquia	Turkey stones.
Piedras de alahona	Mill stone.
Piedras de amolar cuchillos pā zapateros, carpinteros	Shoemakers,' carpenters' hones.
Piedras de vuelta	Grindstones.
Piedras pomez	Pumice stone.
Pieges à rats fer forts (F.)	Strong rat traps.
Piel curtida	Tanned leather.
Pieles lanares, matadero	Sheep skins with wool on, imported from slaughter-house.
Pieles lanares, lavado	Washed skins with wool on.
Pieles lanares, corderito	Lamb skins with wool on.
Pieles lanares, criollo	Young sheep skins with wool on.
Pieles lanares, mestizo	Mixed breed skins with wool on.
Pieles de gamo, tejin, oso, castor conejo	Doe, badger, bear, beaver, rabbit skins.
Piernas de bocados	Cheeks for bits.
Piernas de calceta, piano de	Drawers' leg piano, grand piano.
Pilas pā agua bendita	Fonts for holy water.
Pilderos de varios tamanos	Apothecary's pill pots or jars.
Pilon	Steelyard weight.
Pimienta	Pepper.
Pincelas de pluma	Camels' hair brushes, in quill.
Pincelas de artistas	Artists' pencils.
Pincelas redondas	Sash tools.
Pincelitos cerda blanca	White bristle sash tools.
Pinces fines pour espines (F.)	Tweezers for taking out thorns.
Pinches pā atuzar el coke y avivar el fuego en las chimeneas	Sets fire irons.
Pintada, loza	Painted earthenware.
Pintas menudas, Indianas con	Small spots, regatta prints with.
Pintas y listas varias, loza	Various colours and stripes, earthenware.
Pintas firmes	Fast colours.
Pintura en aceite	Oil paint.
Pintura blanca, amarilla, canaria, colorada verde, azul, negra, &c.	Paint, white, yellow, canary, red, green, blue, black, &c.
Pintura color roble, caoba, &c.	Paint, oak, mahogany colour, &c.

Pinzas pā azucar	Sugar tongs.
Pinzas pā zapateros, &c.	Shoemakers' pincers, &c.
Pinza pā sacar espinas de la grana	Tweezers.
Pinzones de resorte con tubos medianos y pequeños	Spring punches with small and medium bits.
Piñas acero, molinos pā café con	Coffee mills with steel crushers.
Piñon, rueda	Small cog-wheel or pinion.
Pioches, trous ronds (F.)	Picks, round holes, Brazil picks.
Pioches (F.)	Hoes.
Piolilla	Twine.
Piperia	Tubing.
Pique, á cuadritos	Waistcoating, small check.
Piquer doble empedrador	Double pricker.
Piquetillo de empedrador	Macadamiser's picks.
Piquillos de acero fundido	Cast steel points.
Piquois (F.)	Picks.
Pirlanes hierro colado	Cast iron plates.
Pisapapeles	Paper weights.
Piso pā espejo	Looking-glass stands.
Pisos, enloza porcelana pā	Earthenware, flooring tiles.
Pistos pā escopeta	Nipples for guns.
Pistolas giratorias	Revolver pistols.
Pistolas de gancho	Stock pistols.
Pistolas de arzon	Horse pistols.
Pistoleras	Holsters for pistols.
Pistones ò chimeneas pā escopeta	Nipples for guns.
Pistones pā escopeta	Percussion caps.
Piteras ò piteritos pā enfermos	Sick feeders.
Pito de alarma	Alarum whistle.
Pizarras, lapices pā	Slate pencils.
Pizarras, marco de piño	Slates with pinewood frames.
Pizarrines	Slate pencils.
Placas de hierro pā las juntas	Iron chair plates for joining.
Planas pā albañiles	Masons' plastering trowels.
Planas pā tonelero	Hand round shaves.
Planchas y plancas	Sheets of metals, &c.
Planchas hierro angular	Bars angle iron.
Planchas de hierro	Iron sheets.
Planchas bruñidas por un lado, de una cara	Sheets bright on one side.
Planchas de cobre pā clarificadores	Copper sheets for clarificators.
Planchas de cobre pā fondo	Copper bottoms.
Planchas de tola	Sheets Osier bed iron.
Planchas de china pā puertas	China finger plates.
Planchas de metal pā puertas	Brass finger plates.
Planchas pā ropa economicas, de vapor	Sad irons, American box irons.
Planchas huecas	Hollow or box irons.
Planchas pā sombrerero	Hatters' irons.
Planchas de asiento	Chair plates (rail).
Planchas pā cocina	Kitchen sheets or ranges.

Planchas de cobre, de forro	Copper sheets for sheathing.
Planchas pā costado	Copper sheets for sides.
Planchuela hierro	Flat bar iron.
Planchuela de acero pā muelles	Flat bar steel for springs.
Planchuela de empate, pares	Fish bar, pairs.
Planevas pā albañil	Plastering trowels.
Planos, plancos vidrio	Flat glass.
Plantillas pā calentar planchas	Dutch stoves for heating sad irons
Plantillas	Pattern or model.
Plantillos de silla	Railway chairs.
Plata electrica	Electro-plate.
Plata labrada	Worked silver.
Plates, assiettes (F.)	Flat plates.
Plateado	Plated.
Platicos	Small plates.
Platines à anses avec rebord à baguette (F.)	Plates with handle with ring edge.
Platina, botones platina blancos dobles	White metal trouser buttons.
Platina, cucharas de	Plated spoons.
Platinas, hierro	Flat bar iron.
Platilla, cucharas de	Plated spoons.
Platilla, blanco de hilo	White linen Platilla.
Platillo	Flange.
Platillos, llaves de hierro con, tubos con	Iron cocks, tubes with flanges.
Platillos, tazas con	Cups with saucers.
Platillos pā ceniza	Plates for cigar ashes.
Platillos ò Royales	Platillos or royales.
Platinitas hierro dulce	Wrought iron flat bars.
Platitos	Saucers.
Platos llanos, hondos, ovales	Flat, deep, oval dishes.
Platos trinches, cabretilla	Dinner plates, kid pattern.
Platos chicos pā postres	Small dessert plates.
Platos lazo, centro	Plates, lazo centre.
Platos pā jamon	Ham plates.
Platos de retrato y casamiento	Portrait and marriage plates.
Platos de Budin	Pudding plates.
Platos tendidos	Flat plates.
Platos de vapor	Evaporating dishes.
Platos de balanza	Scales.
Platos de lata pā mesa	Tin plate dinner plates.
Platos de estaño	Pewter dinner plates.
Platos de orilla	Edged plates.
Platoncitos	Round deep dishes.
Platones	Dishes.
Plomado de hierro pā albañiles con su nuez de madera	Masons' plummets with wooden wheel.
Plomo en barritas	Lead in bars.
Plomo en lingotes ò galapagos	Lead in pigs or bars.
Plomo calcinado	Lead ashes.

Plomo color	Lead colour.
Plomo en plancha	Lead sheet.
Plumas acero Inglesas pā dibujo tipografico	English steel pens for typographical drawing.
Plumas pā escribir	Writing pens.
Plumas de avestra	Ostrich plumes.
Plumas finas	Fine hearth brushes.
Plumas ó pajas de agua, llaves de bronce pā	Brass cooks for water tubing.
Plugastel	Loom dowlas.
Plugastel de lino	Linen plugastels or dowlas.
Plumbagin de hierro	Iron filings.
Pocillos con platillos pequeños	Chocolate cups and saucers.
Podadera corva	Pruning hook.
Podaderas pā cacao	Cocoa knives.
Podadeiras de ferro (P.)	Unhandled spades.
Poeles à frire (F.)	Frying pans.
Poignées de malles (F.)	Trunk handles.
Polainas de cuero	Leather spatterdashes, antigropeloi gaiters.
Poleas de metal ò ruedas	Brass pulleys.
Poltronas de metal	Brass easy chairs.
Polvora pā barrenos	Blasting powder.
Polvora gruesa de cañon, lustrada y fuerte	Large cannon powder bright and strong.
Polvora mostacilla	Fine grain powder.
Polvoreras	Powder flasks.
Polvorines de asta con cuerdas verdes	Horn powder flasks with green cords.
Polvos hierro pā maquina	Iron powder for machines.
Pomitos tinta negra pā escribir	Small bottles black writing ink.
Pomo del cabo, de un cuchillo, dorado	Knife handles with brass cap.
Pomos de vinagreras	Bottles for cruet frames.
Ponces de volta (P.)	Grass knives.
Ponso, ponzo, hilo	Bright crimson thread.
Porcelanas, tazitas y (Guat.)	Cups and saucers.
Porcelanas, orinales	Chambers.
Porcelanas, hierro dulce, esmaltadas	Enamelled wash basins.
Porcelaine (F.)	China.
Portaplaneados	Box irons.
Portabotellas plateadas	Plated bottle stands.
Porta cuchillos	Knife holders, plate baskets.
Portaplumas	Pen holders.
Portaplumas de palo	Wood pen holders.
Porongos con plato y tapa	Earthenware pitcher with stand and cover.
Porrones de vidrio, tamaño grande	Glass pitcher large size.
Porte regular, azadas	Fair size. hoes.
Portes y carretages	Porterage and carterage.
Posadeiras (P.)	Ladles.

cartuchos con postes pā ca-renado	Patent cartridges for buck shooting
os	Single doors or shutters.
esfericos, cilindricos pā que-carbon animal	Spherical, cylindrical pots for burn-ing animal charcoal.
roja de lata	Tin jacks.
pā cocinar cola	Glue pots.
le repuesto	Spare pots (to replace breakages).
pintura blanca	Iron kegs white paint.
de polvora fina	Fine powder flasks.
e nuit, cuvettes et cruchons	Chambers, wash basins, and ewers.
os con platos	Chocolate cups with saucer.
o (loza)	Pocillo shape.
de negocio	Market price.
amarillos pā escudos de cha-as de maos de fichar (P.)	Yellow escutcheon nails for chest of drawers.
dores pā el pelo	Hair pins.
do, azul, roso, morado	Painted blue, rose, and purple.
do vasos crystal	Pressed glass tumblers.
s pā los corchos de botellas	Presses for corks.
s pa copiar	Copying presses.
s de mano	Hand presses.
s pā sillar papel en seco	Embossing press.
las de botas	Boot laces.
itas pā botines elasticos	Tapes for loops for elastic boots.
era hierro galvanizado	Galvanized iron dripping pans.
l'eau (F.)	Canal, trench, or funnel for supply-ing water.
nes pā los pies	Leg locks.
nes pā pescuezo	Neck collars or locks.
gio de	Patent of.
lla negra	Black prunella.
e madeira con sus mechas (P.)	Wood boring brace with bits.
tenedor 4 puas	Four-prong fork.
ecillas pā violin	Violin bridges.
s registras	Register doors.
s de horno	Furnace doors.
antes, pujabantes	Butteris, paring knives, farriers' knives to cut horses' hoofs.
etes	Watchmakers' pincers.
rios de boj	Box rules.
	Polished.
res pā taco, pā enfranque	Spokeshaves, for the heel, for the waist of boot.
eras, tazas puncheras pā la-las manos y la cara	Wash basins.
eras y jarras largas	Wash basins and tall ewers.
roma, cuchillos con	Dub-point knives.
pā cigarros	Cigar tips.
pā tacos de billar	Tips for billiard cues.

Puntas Paris	Paris points.
Punteras pā talabartero	Saddlers' punches.
Punteros	Stone-cutters' chisels, jumpers.
Puntillas aletinas	Winged points or tacks.
Puntillos	Tacks, points of Paris.
Puntillos sin cabeza pa persianas	Brads or tacks without heads for Venetian blinds.
Puntillas metal pā bocallaves	Brass escutcheon pins.
Puntillas de cobre	Copper pins.
Puntillas sin cabeza pā zapatero	Shoe bills or points.
Puntillas metal con cabeza	Brass headed tacks.
Punto de algodon liso blanco	Plain white cotton lace.
Punto blanco algodon bordado	Embroidered white cotton lace.
Punto, camisas de hilo de punto	Knit linen under shirts.
Punto de escoces de tul liso blanco	White fancy net for curtains, Scotch white plain lace.
Punzo	Crimson, red.
Punzonera	Axle pin.
Punzones de resorte con tubos	Spring punch plyers.
Punzones de presion	A punching machine.
Punzones pā talabartero	Saddlers' punches.
Punzone pā encuadernar	Stationers' awls.
Punzones pā destriar ó perfilar	Punches for fluting soles of shoes.
Puñal	Dagger.
Puño, machetes con	Handled matchets.
Puño de china, resorte con	Latch with china handle.
Puño laton, pā puerta	Brass door handle.

Q

Quatorias, giratorias	Revolvers.
Queba, gueba nozes (P.)	Nut crackers.
Quemado, aceite metal	Boiled oil, annealed metal.
Quemadores de gas	Gas burners.
Quemadores de abanico	Fantail burners.
Queseras	Cheese stands.
Quepies	Military caps.
Queue, à (F.)	Long tail handle.
Quiales	Quirks.
Quijados ò tornillos	Smiths' vices.
Quina	Peruvian bark.
Quinques	Hanging lamps.
Quiribites	Small tue irons.
Quijo	Shaft of engine.
Quita soles, parasoles, sombrillas	Parasols.

R

Rabaneras	Radish dishes.
Rabisa de fuete	Whip thong.
Rabisa, cuchara de albañil rema-chada	Tang of trowel, riveted.

Rabo, asa	Long handle, bow handle.
Rabots (F.)	Smoothing planes.
Raiz, brusas de raiz pā caballo	Bass root horse brushes or dandy brushes.
Rallos pā nuez moscado	Nutmeg graters.
Rallos pā pan	Bread graters.
Ramales de 2 campanas pā cañeria	Branches 2 sockets for pipes.
Ramales de hierro 2 eslabones	Two-link iron leg chains.
Ramillones ó bombones	Sugar bowls or kettles.
Ramo de flores artificiales	Bunch of artificial flowers.
Ranas centrales de chucho triple	Central frogs for triple switch.
Ranas centrales ó laterales	Frogs for railways, central and lateral.
Ranaduras pā carpinteros	Carpenters' grooving planes.
Rancho, cucharones pā	Ladles for mess.
Ranuradores pā carpintero	Grooving planes.
Rapadura	Cane waste.
Rascapies ò rascadores pā botas	Foot, door, scrapers.
Rascardero ò rascador pā caballo	Currycombs.
Rasoirs avec cuirs en etui (F.)	Razors with strops in cases.
Rasoirs manches noires et blanches	Razors, black and white handles.
Raspadores ó escofinas pā igualar, la estaquilla dentro de los zapatos	Rasps for smoothing pegs.
Rasquetas pā caballo con peines	Currycombs with mane combs.
Rasquetas pā tacho, pā buque	Sugar pan scrapers, ship scrapers.
Rastrillo	Hatchet.
Rastro pā jardin	Garden rake.
Ratières (F.)	Rat traps.
Ratoneras de jaulitos pā arrieros	Cage rat traps for carriers.
Ratoneras pā perros "Gibarros"	Rat traps for dogs.
Ratoneras de alambre, de cajon	Wire and box rat traps.
Ratoneras de hierro de cepo, de resorte	Spring rat traps.
Ratoneras de dientes	Teethed rat traps.
Ratoneras de jaula	Cage rat traps.
Ratoneras de raton, Irlandesas	Irish mouse traps.
Ravisa, cabo de	Taper handle.
Raya à raya	Line for line.
Raya, limas de una raya	Single cut files.
Rayado	Scored, fluted.
Rebajadores de tornillo	Screw fillister planes.
Rabotes, ferros pā (P.)	Plane irons.
Rebolve plateado	Plated revolver.
Recamada	Chamber of a gun.
Recambio, boquillas de	Spare bits for punches.
Recocido, alambre	Annealed wire.
Recodos ò Tes pā gas	T's for gas.
Redanchos y ganchos	Ship thimbles and hooks.
Redoblones	Rivets.
Refriaderas	Coolers.
Regaderas pā jardines	Garden watering cans with rosettes.

Regatones metal ochavados	Brass octagon ferrules for walking-sticks.
Reglas de boj, de marfil	Box, ivory rules.
Reglas pantometras	Pantometer rules.
Reglas pā hacer lineas paralelas	Rules for making parallel lines.
Reglas de acanelar con su cuchillo	Plough cutting gauge knife.
Reglas tipos de madera con costillos de metal en sus extremos pā los aparejadores	Standard wooden rules with brass caps at their extremities for overseers.
Reglas metalicas con chanflan blanco, dividas en milimetros con sus cajas	Metallic rules with white bevel, divided into millimeters, with their cases.
Reglas pā reglar papel	Rules for ruling paper.
Regular, calidad	Middle quality.
Reguladores	Regulators (elec. tel.)
Rejas de Isleña	Teneriffe ploughshares.
Rejas pā arado	Ploughshares.
Rejas de cubo	Socket ploughshares.
Rejas con su aro y agujero	Ploughshares with ring and hole in the socket.
Rejadas pā arado	Plough paddles or spuds.
Rejadas de bara ó vara pā limpiar arados	Plough paddles to clean ploughshares.
Rejilla, bandas china de	Netted bandas or sashes.
Rejillas encuadradas de relex	Square grates, bevilled edge.
Rejillas pā fogon	Grates for stoves.
Rejillas	Brackets for shelves.
Rejillas hierro pā celosias	Wove wire for windows.
Relej, relex por dentro	Bevelled edge inside.
Relieve, platos granito aguila	Relief granite eagle plates.
Rellano,-a	Landing of staircase.
Rellena ó macisa, asa pā tazas	Solid tea cup handles.
Relox de faltriquera	Watch.
Relox de pared	House clock.
Relox con despertador	Alarm clock.
Relox, savoneta	Hunting watch.
Relox oro pā señora con sus tapas	Ladies' gold hunting watch.
Relojes del sol	Sun dials.
Relojes pā asar	Brass bottle jacks.
Relojitos	Small watches.
Remachado, ojo de pala	Shovel eye, rivetted.
Remaches pā pailas	Boiler or sugar pan rivets, flat heads
Remaches de cobre chiquitos con arandelitas	Small copper rivets with washers.
Remaches hierro prensados pā hormas	Pressed iron sugar funnel rivets.
Remaches hierro, cobre pā calderos de vapor	Iron, copper steam boiler rivets.
Remate	Auction sale.
Remates pā cama	Bed ornaments.
Remates de puertas	Door fasteners.

Remates dorados	Gilt mountings as of fire irons.
Remillones, de cobre, de hierro estañado	Copper, tinned iron bowls for sugar estates.
Rempujos pā marinero, montados en cuero	Sailors' palms, mounted in leather.
Repartideras, repartidores con cruzeta	Parting bowls with cross.
Repartideras hierro estañado pā ingenio	Sugar estate parting bowls.
Repisa	Shelf, bracket, or pedestal.
Replanes	Jack planes.
Repuestos de diferentes dimensiones pā taladro	Spare pieces, different sizes, for punching machine.
Resfriaderas,-ores, ò gavetas	Sugar coolers.
Resguardos de fuego	Fenders.
Resina elastica	Gutta percha.
Resmas trapo de lija	Reams glass paper.
Resones pā embarcaciones pequeñas	Small anchors, kedge anchors.
Resorte de seda pā botines	Silk elastic web for boots.
Resorte, punzones de	Spring punches.
Resorte, balancitas de	Small spring balances.
Rosortes pā mesa	Table springs, or catches.
Resortes ò semicirculos pā escritorio	Quadrants, catches, or half circles, for counting house doors.
Ressorts à boudin (F.)	Girdles, bracelets, or African coils.
Retenidas	Martingales.
Retortas	Retorts.
Retrancos pā ferro carril	Railway breaks.
Retrifla, retrilla, retrillia, retillia	Coffee huskers.
Reverberos amarillos	Reflectors or street lamps.
Reves por dentro, por fuera, gurbias	Bevelled inside, outside gouges.
Revocar, cucharas pā	Plasterers' trowels.
Revuelo, fleco	Double flounce.
Ribeteado, la boca de los codos ribeteada	The mouth of the elbows, rimmed, hemmed, rivetted.
Riendas redondas con crucero y flecos	Round reins with cross face pieces and fringes, or nose piece, or band
Riendas simples y dobles	Single and double reins.
Riendas, cabezadas con sus	Leather heads with reins.
Riendas, jarcia cañamo pā hacer	Hemp rope for making plough lines.
Rifles, pistolas	Rifled pistols.
Rivete	Edging or border.
Rizar, maquina pā rizar ropa	A goffering machine.
Rizadores pā ropa	Goffering irons.
Roble, pintado	Painted oak colour.
Rodajas de laton	Brass castors.
Rodajas pā espuelas	Spur rowels.
Rodillos pā hilera	Small steel rollers for a mint.
Roldanas, una rueda pā lamparas	One wheel lamp pulleys.
Roldanas pā cama, pā sofa	Castors, for bedstead or sofa.
Roldanas de espiga pā pies de mesa	Castors for table feet, with spike.

Roldanas pā vidriera	Sash pulleys or rollers.
Roldanas hierro de patente, cilindro de bronce	Iron pulley wheels with brass cylinders or bushes.
Roldanas de hierro	Block iron sheaves.
Roldanas de cabilla	Moveable castors.
Roldanas pā embutir	Flush castors.
Roldanas de planchuelas	Flange wheels and plates.
Roldanas de barras chatas	Wheels and plates flanged.
Roldanas de barras redondas	Wheels and plates grooved.
Roldanas de goma pā tubos	India rubber washers for tubes.
Roldanas de cabilla pā secadero ò gaveta	Wheels and plates for round iron for sugar dryer.
Roldanas con sus cajuelas pā girar sobre cabilla	Wheels and plates for running on round iron.
Rolletas pā clavar pā zapatero	Shoemakers' small wheels for nailing work.
Rollo ò rollado pā jardin	Garden roll.
Rollos de laton en plancha	Rolls of sheet brass.
Rollos, jarcia pita de manila	Coils or rolls Manilla rope.
Roma, punta	Dub point.
Romanas de muelle hechura de reloj	Steelyard, with watch shape spring.
Romanas de palanca y pilon	Steelyards with lever and ball.
Romanas de pilon con gancho	Steelyard with ball, weight and hook
Romanas de plata forma, sobre ruedas	Platform steelyard, or weighing machine on wheels.
Romanitas de canuto pā el bolsillo	Small pocket steelyards.
Romero	Rosemary colour.
Rondanas	Wheels and plates.
Rondanas con armazon	Pulleys with blocks for wells.
Rondanas, rondanitas	Pulleys for hanging lamps.
Roperos	Wardrobes.
Rosa, rosado	Rose or pink.
Rosaces assorties (F.)	Rosettes assorted.
Roscas de prision con llave pā pie	Leg locks with key.
Roscas de prisiones pā pescuezo con su cadena	Neck locks with chain.
Rosetas pulidas	Bright spur rowels.
Rotulo, sobre tarjeta	Inscription on label, or label.
Royales ó platillos,-as	Royals or platillos.
Royales de lino blanco	White linen royals, or linen creas.
Royales de algodon blanco, negro	White, black cotton royals or platillos.
Royales café oscuro, aplomado	Dark, lead colour royals or platillos
Rozaderas pā piña	Pine bills.
Ruan de algodon	Cotton ruan.
Rueda de molino, de respeto	Mill wheel, spare wheel.
Rueda de aumento	Fly, increasing, or multiplying wheel.
Rueda pā carro de mula, pā volante	Mule cart, fly or gig wheel.
Rueda Catalina	Spur, cog, or catalina wheel.
Rueda Catarina	Large cog bevel wheel on perpendicular shaft for giving the motion.

Rueda conica dentada	Bevel cog wheel.
Rueda piñon	Small cog wheel.
Rueda farol ó corona	Lantern or crown wheel.
Rueda, brazos, serohas, y budares	Wheel with arms, rim segments and centre plates.
Ruibarbo	Rhubarb.
Rusias de lino blanco, hilo grueso	White Russian sheeting, strong thread.
Rusias Belgas ó Inglesas	Belgian or English sheeting.
Rusias de lino blanco	Russian creas.

S

Sabana	Sheet.
Sable, cabo de asta	Horn handled sword or matchett.
Sable pã marina, pã caballeria	Swords for the navy, for cavalry.
Saboneta, relox de oro	Gold hunting watch.
Sacabocados de golpe, de talabarteros	Saddlers' punches.
Sacabocados con sus pistones	Punches with bits.
Sacabocados de tenaza	Punch pliers.
Sacabotas	Boot jacks.
Saca brocas	Tack drawers.
Sacamuelas	Tooth drawers.
Sacatornillos	Turnscrews.
Sacatrapos	Wadworms, or ramrod screws.
Saccarolha (P.)	Patent corkscrew with rack.
Sachos picos	Spades or Brazil picks.
Sachos (Bucharest)	Common spades.
Sachos (Central America)	Bread graters.
Sacos de noche	Carpet bags.
Sacos pã café	Coffee bags.
Sacos de yute doble y tupido	Very stout jute sacks.
Safras pã ferreiro (P.)	Smiths' anvils.
Sal en granel, en grano	Rough salt.
Sal amoniaco	Ammoniac salt.
Sal de Inglaterra, sulfato de magnesia	Epsom salt, sulphate of magnesia.
Sal de espuma	Fine salt.
Sala, escupideras de	Drawing room spittoons.
Saladas	Salt pits.
Salados	Salting places.
Salampores	Salampores, or china mantas.
Saleas pã galapagos	Rugs for saddles.
Saleros	Salt cellars.
Salseras con sus fuentes	Sauce boats and stands.
Salta reglas	Sliding rules.
Salteadas, agujas	Synoptical ground sharps, needles.
Salteados, los agujeros que no sean	The holes not to be zig zag or in and out.
Salvaderas	Sand boxes.
Salvavidas	Life preservers.

Salvillas ó compoteras con pies	Sweetmeat dishes with feet.
Sandalos lustrados ó lustrosos, labrados	Glazed lining, embossed, figured sandalos.
Sandalos de lustre negro liso pā forro	Lustre sandalos (silesias) plain black for lining.
Sandalos de algodon liso, tejido asargado	Plain twilled cotton sandalos.
Sandalos cotonados	Sandals.
Sangre de drago	Brown varnished.
Sarampora, sarampor, ó manta de china	Sarampores, imitation of Chinese manta.
Sarazas	Cotton prints, chintz.
Sarga	Serge.
Sarta de cuentas	String of beads,
Sartenes	Frying pans.
Savoneta	Hunting watch.
Scies á rases (F.)	Iron-back saws.
Scies á cran d'acier fondu (F.)	Cast steel rib saws with handles.
Scies dites taureaux pour troncer, à dents droites (F.)	Saws called bulls, for cutting trunks, straight teeth.
Sebo pā eje	Cart grease.
Seda pura, pañuelones de	Corahs, all silk.
Segaderas	Breast straps.
Seguetas	Back hand saws.
Seguitos tela metalica pā cafeteras	Brass wove wire bags for coffee pots.
Segura pā carpintero	Carpenters' axe.
Seguretas pā tonelero	Coopers' axes.
Seisabado	Sexagon.
Sellos de cartas	Letter seals.
Semanario de navajas	Seven day razor case.
Sencillo	Light or single.
Sentaderas pā planchas	Sad iron stands.
Sepia	Sepia colour.
Serga	Serge.
Seringas de bomba	Enemas.
Seron de grana	A frail of cochineal.
Seron ó seretas de arroz	A large sack in which a number of bags full may be put, for rice.
Serrotes pā dar vuelto, de voltear	Key hole saws.
Serrotes de trozar	Cross cut saws.
Serruchos de mano	Hand saws.
Serruchos de mano pā podar café	Hand saws for pruning coffee.
Serruchos de calar, con punta	Compass saws, pointed.
Serruchos de trozar	Cross-cut saws.
Serruchos de armar	Web saws.
Serruchos oberduguillos	Key hole saws.
Serruchos de costilla ó lomo, de hierro ó de metal	Iron or brass back saws, tenon saws.
Serruchos de espejo, dientes muy finos, hoja doble y reforzada	Mirror polished hand saws, teeth very fine, double strong blade.
Serrures pour armoires (F.)	Cupboard locks.

Serrures de malles (F.)	Trunk locks.
Servicios de loza de mesa	Dinner services.
Servicios pă café y tè	Tea and coffee services.
Servicios pă trinchar	Pairs carvers.
Servicios altos con tapa blancos	White deep chair pans with covers.
Servicios de cama	Bed pans.
Servicios de pala	Bidet pans, French shape.
Servicios de hierro dulce con tapas	Wrought iron bidet pans with covers
Servilletas de mesa	Table napkins.
Servilleteros	Napkin rings.
Sierra de vuelo grande con bastidor pă sacar tablas	Large pit saws with frames for cutting planks.
Sierras de aire con armazon ó manigueta	Pit saws with boxes and tillers, or handles.
Sierras cabrillas	Pit saws.
Sierras tromsadoras pă cortar arboles gruesos	Cross-cut saws to cut thick trees.
Sierras de continuar	Continuous band saws.
Sierras circulares	Circular saws.
Sierras de verduguillo, de calar, dientes finos, hoja delgada	Compass saws, fine teeth, thin blade.
Sierras de redondear, de rodear, de voltear, pă armaduras, de armar, de brazo, angostas	Saw webs, web saws, or key hole saws.
Sierras de costilla, de verduguillo	Narrow back saws.
Sierras de ajustar	Adjusting saws.
Sierras pă abrir	Fret saws.
Sierras cola de raton	Rat tail saws.
Sierras de espejo	Mirror polished saws.
Silbato	Whistle.
Silesias	Silesias, (drapery).
Sillas, poltronas	Chairs, arm chairs.
Sillas de estremidad de chucho	Chairs for end of switch (rail).
Sillas con rejilla	Chairs with open seat.
Sillas lisas cuero de chancho, de cochino	Plain hogskin saddles.
Sillas, colchadas de montar	Quilted riding saddles.
Sillas de montar habilitadas	Saddles with saddle cloth and double bridle, or with all requisites.
Silleria, pilares de	Pillars of masonry.
Silleros	Saddlers.
Sillitas papier maché pă iglesia	Small papier mache chairs for churches.
Sillones mecedores, forros de tafilete punzo	Rocking chairs, red morocco covers.
Sillones ò butacas	Arm chairs.
Sillones con respaldo de alfombra	Chairs with carpet furniture.
Sobre caja de oro	Gold watch case.
Sobre cama	Counterpane.
Sobre cinchas	Overgirths.
Sobre mesas	Table covers.

Sobres pà cartas	Letter envelopes.
Soda seco y en polvo	Dry soda ash, pure alkali
Sofa, alfombras ò estrillas pā	Sofa rugs or mats.
Sofas de hierro	Iron benches for public promenades.
Soga de cañamo	Hemp rope.
Soldadores de cobre	Copper soldering irons.
Soldadura, metal, fina, gorda	Brass solder, fine, coarse.
Sombra de Italia	Raw umber.
Sombreros de cuero con su tranca	Hat boxes with lock.
Sombreros de chimenea	Chimney pots.
Sombreros de felpa	Felt hats.
Sombreros de paja	Straw hats.
Sommier elastique (F.)	Spring mattress.
Sondas	Plummets.
Soperas con tapa, plato ó bandeja, y cucharon	Soup tureens, with cover, stand, and ladle.
Soperas de lata	Tin plate soup tureens.
Soperitos	Sauce tureens.
Soperos petits avec couvercles et cuillers (F.)	Small soup or sauce tureens with covers and ladles.
Soperos	Soup plates, sometimes soup tureens
Sopletes	Blow pipes.
Sortijas de oro	Gold rings.
Sosa caustica	Caustic soda.
Sotrozos de chavetas pā carreta	Plate wagon cotter pins.
Sotrozos pā volantes	Gig cotter or lynch pins.
Sovellas ou sovelas pā pontiar (P.)	Stitching awls.
Sovellas aplazar, direitas (P.)	Stabbing awls, straight.
Suaves, limas planas	Flat smooth files.
Suaves, limas media	Half smooth files.
Suavizadores	Razor strops.
Subido, color, precio	Deep in colour, high in price.
Sudaderas ò paños pā silla	Saddle cloths, sweat dryers.
Suela Inglesa pā bombas	English leather for pumps.
Suela planchuela	Pressed sole leather.
Suela sencilla	Light sole leather.
Suela curtida pā zapatos	Tanned leather for soles of shoes.
Suela de cuero doble pā bombas	Tanned thick leather for pumps.
Suela de lazo	White lace.
Suelas charoladas, fuertes y grandes	Strong and large japanned hides for aprons.
Suelto	Loose.
Sufridores pā guijos	Shaft drivers, stays for shaft centres
Sufridores con espiga cuadrada	Centres with square spike.
Sumidero	Sewer, sink.
Suncho en el furo	Hoop on the nozzle.
Sunchos, hierro pā	Iron for hoops, or hoop iron.
Sunchos de carros	Tyres for carts.
Superficie de rotacion	Rolling surface.
Surtido, un	An assortment.

T

Tabaquera	Snuff box.
Tablas reales	Backgammon tables.
Tablas, limas	Flat files.
Tableros de suela figura de libro de ajedrez	Folding book shape, leather, draft, chess boards.
Taburetes, tornillos pä	Stool or chair screws.
Tachos, tachitos	Sugar pans, small.
Tachos al vacio con muñones	Vacuum sugar pans with lugs or ears.
Tachos pä raciones	Small pans for rations.
Tachuelas de hierro, azuladas, bruñidas	Blued, bright, iron tacks, brads.
Tachuelas aforradas	Coated tacks.
Tachuelas de cobre, pä militar	Copper tacks, military copper tacks.
Tachuelas de oro pä sillas, amarillas, ó doradas	Gold colour chair nails.
Tacisas, tacises, ò aguinches	Tacises matchets, bill hooks.
Tacitas con asa y platos	Small handled cups and saucers.
Tacon de zapato, taco	Heel of shoe.
Tacos, punzones pä	Gun wads, punches for.
Tacos pä señoras	Ladies' billiard cues.
Tafilete, marneco, asiento de	Morocco seat.
Tafiletes pä sombreros	Skins or skivers for hats.
Tahona pä moler trigo	Wheat mill.
Tairières, tarières (F.)	Screw augers.
Tajaderas pä cortar barras de hierro	Chisels for cutting iron bars.
Talabartero	Saddler.
Talabarteria, instrumentos de	Saddlers' tools.
Taladros con mechas	Braces with bits.
Taladros	Drill mining bars.
Taladros salamonicos	Auger drills.
Taladros con repuestos de diferentes dimensiones	Punching machine or drilling machine with spare pieces of different sizes.
Talcos pä faroles	Sheets of horn or horn leaves for lanterns.
Talladores	Turners.
Talleres de mesa	Cruet stands.
Tambor pä limpiar	Lap machine for cleaning.
Tambores pä cafè	Coffee roasters.
Tambores de trapiche, corona pä	Sugar mill rolls, cog wheels for.
Tanques bajos y altos	Low and tall mugs.
Tanques dorados, loza	Gold lustre mugs.
Tanques altos	Tall tankard mugs.
Tanques de hierro	Iron tanks.
Tanques pä enfriar azucar	Tanks for cooling sugar.
Tanques ó cristalizadores pä azucar	Tanks or sugar crystallizers.
Tapacetes de carruages	Carriage or gig aprons.
Tapacomidas, tela de alambre	Blued iron wove wire dish covers.

Tapaderas, fuentes pā piezas grandes con sus	Dishes for large joints with their covers.
Tapas sueltas, escupideras pā sala con	Drawing room spittoons with loose covers.
Tapas de tejido de alambre	Wove wire dish covers.
Tapas hierro colado de chumaceras	Glands of washers.
Taperolas de hierro	Iron scuppers.
Tapiceria	Tapestry.
Tapiceros, martillos pā	Upholsterers' hammers.
Tapon	A cork, a plug.
Tarifs (F.)	Pattern books.
Tarières, tarrières à vis avec anneau (F.)	Screw-eyed augers.
Tarières, tarrières à cuillers (F.)	Shell augers.
Tarières, tarrières, à vrilles, à douille	Screw-eyed augers.
Tarières, tarrières à cuillers, à douille	Shell-eyed augers.
Tarjeta, tarjete de pergamio	Parchment labels.
Tarjetera	Card case.
Tarnabilas,-villas de metal pā puertas	Brass door buttons for opening or shutting on plates.
Tarracillas pā azucar	Sugar tongs.
Tarrajas con dados	Screw plates, screw boxes and taps, stocks and dies.
Tarrajas de 1 ò 2 manos	One hand or double hand screw plates.
Tarrajas con sus machos y dados	Screw plates with their males and sets of dies.
Tarrajas pā herrero	Blacksmiths' screw stocks and dies.
Tarrajas completas con sus cajas	Cases stocks and dies complete.
Tarrajitas	Small screw plates, or stocks and dies.
Tarrajitas finas pā platero	Fine screw plates for silversmiths.
Tarro, machetes cabo de	Horn handled matchets.
Tarro, bruñido	Polished horn.
Tarros enteros, medios, de cerveza	Stone quarts, pints, of ale.
Tarros de betun	Bottles of blacking.
Tarros de pintura	Kegs of paint.
Tarteras hierro con sus platos	Cooking pans with plates.
Tarugo	Plug.
Tas pā platero	Silversmiths' anvil.
Tauretes, tavoretes, tornillos pā	Stool screws, same as cot screws.
Tazas calderas, pā caldo	Broth bowls.
Tazas bolas	Bowls, basins, Grecian bowls.
Tazas con espiga de trigo	Teas with ear of wheat in relief.
Tazas con asa y platos ó platillos	Handled cups and saucers.
Tazas de retrato	Portrait teas.
Tazas de almuerzo	Breakfast cups.
Tazas de cintura	Waist shaped cups and saucers.
Tazas pā niños, de paladeo	Teas for children or toy teas.
Tazas platillos, calderas de lustre	Irish cups and saucers.
Tazas de china, pintadas y meladas	China teas painted and dipped.

Tazas de pozillo	Chocolate cups.
Tazitas con oreja	Handled tea cups.
Tazones	Bowls, globe bowls.
Té ó thé	Tea.
Té	T or tee (gasfittings.)
Tejas lisas galvanizadas, con canales, caballetes, grampas clavos y tornillos	Plain galvanized iron tiles, with gutters, ridge caps, staples, nails, and screws.
Tejas acanaladas sin grampas	Corrugated iron tiles without clips or screws.
Tejas pintadas de colorado	Painted red tiles.
Tejido asargado	Weaving twilled.
Tejido de alambre	Wove wire.
Tela pã calcar dibujos	Tracing cloth.
Tela metalica	Wove wire.
Tela real de hilo de colores	Royal cotton or thread cloth.
Tela metalica de laton pã centrifugales	Brass wove wire for centrifugals.
Telas mejoradas	Improved looms.
Teleras pã arado	Plough pins.
Templado, cuchillos triple temple	Tempered, treble tempered knives.
Tenacillas, tenacitas, tenazas, pã azucar	Sugar tongs.
Tenacillas pã platero	Silversmiths' pincers or pliers.
Tenacillas pã rizar ropa	Goffering irons, or small pincers to crimp clothes.
Tenazas de punzon con 8 punzones	Punch pincers with 8 punches.
Tenazas 3 tamaños por el uso de las fraguas	Tongs 3 sizes for the use of forges.
Tenazas pã fragua de herrero	Blacksmiths' pincers.
Tenazas cortantes al lado pã campanilleros	Side cutting pincers or pliers for bell hangers.
Tenazas pã carpintero	Carpenters' pincers.
Tenazas pã albeitares	Pincers for veterinary surgeons.
Tenazas pã herradores	Shoeing pincers.
Tenazas pã cortar	Cutting nippers.
Tenazas pã quemadores de gas	Gas pliers.
Tenazas bruñidas	Bright pliers.
Tendidas, gurbias	Long gouges.
Tendidos, platos	Flat plates.
Tendidos, caneria, cumbreras canales	Lengths of piping, ridge caps, guttering.
Tenedor, pã ostra	Fork, oyster fork.
Teodolito olometrico otaquimetrico	Elometrical tachymetrical theodolite
Tercerola	Carbine.
Tercio	Bale
Terciopelo de algodon, de seda	Cotton, silk velvet.
Tercon	Tierce.
Terebentino,-a	Turpentine.
Terrajas con troqueles y llaves	Screw plates with dies and keys.
Terron, tiza en, añil en terroncitos	Lump chalk, indigo in cakes.

Teteras de plaqué	Plated tea pots.
Tibores pintados y melados	Painted and dipped chambers.
Tibores esmaltados de hierro dulce	Enamelled wrought iron chambers.
Tierra Romana pā suelos	Roman cement or earth for floors.
Tijeras con corte à la derecha pā hoja lateros	Shears for tinmen with edge on the right.
Tijeras pā atusar yeguas	Scissors for clipping horses.
Tijeras pā jardin	Garden scissors.
Tijeras pā uñas y costura	Nail and sewing scissors.
Tijeras pā sastre	Tailors' scissors.
Tijeras pā bordar	Embroidery scissors.
Tijeras pā cortar hoja de lata	Scissors to cut tin plate.
Tijeras pā trasquilar de resorte	Sheep shears with spring.
Tijeras pā esquilar carneros, marca oveja	Trimming scissors.
Tijeras de comba	Bent scissors.
Tijeras límpias pā mostrador	Clean counter scissors.
Tijeras pā pelugueros, pā cortar el pelo	Barbers' or haircutters' scissors.
Tijeras pā atusar mulas	Scissors for clipping mules.
Tijeras corta uñas	Nail scissors.
Tijeras pā parras	Vine scissors.
Tijeras de luz pā tusar	Luz clipping scissors.
Tijeras grandes pā barberos	Barbers' large scissors.
Tijeras pā ojalar	Button hole scissors.
Tijeras de luz sin puntas pā pelugueros de tamaño à proposito	"Luz" scissors for haircutters, without points and suitable size.
Tijeras ó tijeritas de resorte con navajitas	Scissor knives.
Tilles, (F.)	Hammer axes, blued adzes.
Tilles à clous (F.)	Axe hammers for rails.
Timon	Shaft of vehicle.
Tinajas, tinajes	Water jars.
Tinas pā pies	Foot baths.
Tinas ovaladas	Foot baths or wash pans, oval.
Tincar	Borax.
Tinta pā escribir, de japan	Japan writing ink.
Tinta pā duplicar, pā copiar	Copying ink.
Tinta pā imprimir	Printing ink.
Tinta de china, parda negra	Chinese ink, grey and black.
Tinteros de vidrio con pico	Glass inks with lips.
Tinteros de peltre, de carton	Pewter, papier mache ink stands.
Tintilla pā zapateros, pā botas	Blacking for shoemakers, for boots.
Tinto	Claret colour, port wine colour.
Tira de cuero pā coser correa	Leather lace for sewing banding.
Tira de lona	Strip of sail cloth.
Tira de correa de goma	Length of India rubber banding.
Tirabillas de metal	Brass buttons.
Tirabotas	Boot hooks.
Tirabudores de martillo pā sierras de aire	Hammer pit saw sets.

Tirabuzones con arandela	Corkscrews with bars.
Tirabuzones de doblez	Folding corkscrews.
Tirabuzones de escobilla	Corkscrew with brush.
Tirabuzones de bolsa	Pocket corkscrews.
Tirabuzones con corta alambre	Champagne cutters.
Tiraderas pā comodas	Handles for commodes.
Tiraderas pā carretas	Wagon chains.
Tiraderas de cadena con sus grampas	Wagon chains with their hooks.
Tiradores de vidrio à plata	Ornaments or knobs, glass or silver.
Tiradores pā barril	Coopers' vices.
Tirafondos rosca de madera	Wood screws.
Tirafondos pā tonelero	Coopers' drivers, vices.
Tirantes ó tiros pā carro	Trace chains.
Tirantes pā calzones	Braces.
Tirantes pā botes	Boat hooks.
Tiro	Length.
Tiron ou detente de fusil (F.)	Trigger of a gun.
Tiros de espada	Sword belts.
Tiros de lona de 2 cantos	Canvass girth with 2 selvedges.
Tisa, tiza en cascos	Chalk, whitening in casks.
Tisa, tiza ò yeso en piedra	Pipeclay or chalk in pieces.
Tizonero y tenazas	Poker and tongs.
Toallas, tohallas, de alemanisco, de lino	Damask, linen, towels.
Toberas pā fuelles	Bellows' pipes.
Tocador, juegos pā	Toilet table, toilet sets.
Tolas de hierro	Sheet iron.
Toldo, argollas pā	Awning rings.
Tolvas de molinos	Hoppers of mills.
Toneles	Hogsheads, casks or barrels.
Torneiras (P.)	Cocks for boilers.
Tornilladores	Turnscrews.
Tornillos de buey	Ox rings.
Tornillos de cochino	Pig rings.
Tornillos y tuercas pā carruage	Coach screws and nuts.
Tornillos metal pā tachos	Brass screws for sugar pans.
Tornillos con sus tuercas pā mordazas	Screws with nuts for fish bars.
Tornillos pā llanta de carreta	Wagon tyre screws.
Tornillos pā rueda de volante	Gig wheel screws.
Tornillos ò tirafondos roscas de madera, cabeza cuadrada	Wood screws, square heads.
Tornillos pā atar bueyes	Ring swivels for fastening oxen.
Tornillos de ferrocarril ò carriles	Railway bolts.
Tornillos hierro galvanizado	Galvanized iron screws.
Tornillos pā embutir, cabeza de embutir, de encarne	Countersunk headed screws.
Tornillos pā catres, pā cama	Cot, bedstead screws.
Tornillos pā escopetas	Gun screw tips.

Tornillos rosca francesa ò punta de barrena	Screws French thread, or gimlet point.
Tornillos pour un train de laminoirs &c. (F.)	Screws and boxes or housings for confirming and regulating rolls.
Tornillos de bisagras	Hinge screws.
Tornillos pā tocadores	Brass fasteners for sashes.
Tornillos de bronce pā tachos ⸱	Brass screws for sugar pans.
Tornillos con tuercas pā pailas	Screws with nuts for sugar pans.
Tornillos de jaquimon, pā jaquima	Swivel rings or 2-ring swivels.
Tornillos en corne	Tapering or countersunk screws.
Tornillos de presion,	Cramps.
Tornillos de mano con mango	Hand vices with handle.
Tornillos con macho y rosca de bronce	Smiths' vices with male and brass screw.
Tornillos grandes negros	Heavy black vices.
Tornillos con abrazadera en vez de cuña	Vices with clasp or holder instead of wedge cotter key.
Tornillos pā banco ó mesa de herrero	Smiths' bench vices.
Tornillos con hembra de bronce ò metal	Vices with brass box.
Torninhos de mao (P.)	Bright handvices.
Torniquetes	Bill cranks.
Tornos pā herrero	Smiths' vices.
Tornos pā mesa acerados	Steel faced bench vices.
Tornos pā levantar pesos	Lifting jacks or cranes.
Tornos	Turning lathes.
Tornos pequeños pā pulir	Small polishing lathes.
Toros ò sierras pā trozar	Cross-cut saws.
Torteras de lata	Tin baking pans.
Tortillas	Rice bowls.
Trabadeiras (P)	Saw sets.
Trabadores mejorados	Improved saw sets.
Trabadores de martillo pā sierra	Hammer saw sets.
Trabas con cadenas pā caballo	Fetters with chains for horses, horse hobbles.
Trabucos, trabujos trombones	Blunderbusses.
Trados	Tap borers.
Trajes	Dresses.
Trajilla pā jardin	Garden roller.
Trampas de dientes pā ratones, topas	Rat and mole traps with teeth.
Trampas pā ratoncitos	Mouse traps.
Tranchets (F.)	Shoemakers' knives.
Tranchoirs (F.)	Chisels.
Trapantes	Venetian blinds.
Trapiche	Sugar mill and mill for crushing ore.
Trapiche con tambores pā las mazas, guijos, coronas, chumaceras, dados, trompos, sotrozos, arandelas y pernos	Sugar mill, with rollers, shafts, cog wheels, spindle bearers, dies or plates, centres, cotter pins, washers and bolts.

Trapiche con mazas y ruedas de engranage ò dientes correspondieudientes, medias lunas, &c., de laton	Sugar mill with rollers, corresponding cog wheels, half-moons, &c., or brass.
Trapo de papel	Glass paper.
Trapo de lija de vidrio	Glass cloth.
Trapo de lija de esmeril	Emery cloth.
Traquenards Anglais (F.)	English rat traps.
Trasportador de angulos del circulo entero con nonis ò nonio	Transferrer of angles of entire circle with nonis.
Trasquilar, tijeras på	Clipping scissors.
Trencilla de lana	Worsted braid.
Trencilla arqueada ancha	Wide wavy braid.
Trenes de ingenio	Sugar works.
Trepanos	Trepans.
Trillar, maquina på	Threshing machine.
Trinchas,-es de cubo	Socket chisels.
Trinchas de torneros, de tornear	Turners' chisels.
Trinchas de espiga	Firmer chisels.
Trinchas de bocamango	Long socket chisels.
Trinchas på cortar hierro frio	Chisels to cut cold iron.
Trinchas på meter los aros de pipas	Chisels for putting hoops on pipes.
Trinchantes på aves, cabos de asta con guarda	Game carvers, horn handled with guard.
Trinchantes på carne	Meat carvers.
Trinches, plata albata	Albata forks.
Trinches y cuchillos	Forks and spoons.
Trinche, platos de	Fork or flat plates.
Trinchetes på zapatero	Shoemakers' paring knives.
Trinchuelitos de cañon de pluma y pelo camello	Camels' hair pencils, quill tube.
Tripa de cerradura	Inside of lock.
Tripodes	Trivets.
Triscadores, limas pa afilar sierras	Files for sharpening saws.
Trituradores mejorados	Improved sugar crushers.
Trompacitas de boca	Small jews-harp.
Trompas, de lengueta, de laton på muchachos	Jews-harps for boys.
Trompo, plomadas figura de	Top shape plummets.
Trompos de guijos	Centres for shafts.
Trompos con espiga cuadrada	Centres with square spike.
Troquel	Die.
Troza	Piece of trunk of tree.
Truellas, trullas på albañil	Masons' trowels.
Truelles à maçon (F.)	Masons' trowels.
Trujal	Oil mill.
Tuberia på gas	Gas piping.
Tubo, formones de	Socket chisel.
Tubos ó vidrios	Glass chimneys.
Tubos alimentarios på maquina de vapor	Feed pipes for steam engine.
Tubos hierro colado, fundido	Cast iron pipes.

Tubos con platillo	Flange pipes.
Tubos de embudo	Pipes with socket.
Tubos con 2 bocinas ó campanas	Tubes with 2 sockets.
Tubos de codo	Elbows.
Tubos de zinc	Tubes or pipes of zinc.
Tubos pā purgar azucar	Tubes for purifying sugar.
Tubos de punzon	Bits for punches.
Tubos fulminantes	Percussion caps.
Tuercas pā tornillos	Nuts for screws.
Tuercas ó empates pā tubos de gas	Nuts or connections for gas tubes.
Tumbilla, cama con	Bedstead with arrangements for mosquito curtains.
Tupido, manta muy tupida	Very thick or stout manta.
Tusar, tijeras pā	Clipping scissors, or sheep shears.

U

Uniones	Unions, joints, sockets or thimbles.
Unito ò lustre pā botas	Blacking.
Untras car pregos (P.)	Tack drawers.
Uña, pasadores de	Flush bolts.
Uñas, resones de 5	Anchors of 5 claws.
Uñas de taladrar	Centre bits.
Urdidores	Warpers, or warping mills.
Urina plateada	Plated urn.
Uso de familia	Familias, shirting.
Uso merino, imitacion	Imitation merino style.
Utensiles pā ingenio	Sugar estate utensils.
Utiles de carpinteria, pā jardin	Carpenters', garden tools.
Utiles pā dar barrenas	Blasting tools.
Utiles.	Tools of every kind.

V

Vaceado, hierro	Cast iron.
Vacias pā barbero	Barbers' basins.
Vajilla ordinaria de porcelana	Ordinary china dinner service.
Valvulas	Valves or plugs.
Valvulas de seguridad doble	Strong safety valves.
Valvulas de retencion y tubo	Stop or inlet and outlet valves with tube.
Valvulas de parar el vapor, caja de	Valve to stop or give off steam, case for.
Vanda, platos de vanda azul	Plates with blue band.
Vara de medir, de burgos	Spanish yard measure.
Vara de boj angosta ou estreita (P.)	Narrow box rules.
Vara de cortina	Curtain rod.
Vara de carruage	Coach shaft.
Varilla de hierro	Iron nail strip, small bars.
Varilla dorada	Gilt beading.
Varilla bruñida de laton	Polished brass rods.
Varillita	Rod iron.

Vasijas	Vessels.
Vasijas pä barbero, de loza, de laton	Earthenware, brass, barbers' basins.
Vasitos de licor	Small liqueur glasses.
Vasos de vidrio, lisos	Plain glass tumblers.
Vasos moldados	Moulded tumblers.
Vasos de cristal prensado	Pressed glass tumblers.
Vasos de loza con oreja	Earthenware mugs with handle.
Vasos pä vino, licores, &c.	Small glasses, for wine, liqueurs, &c.
Vassouras, vazouras (P.)	Bass brooms, hearth brushes.
Vazadores de mola (P.)	Spring punch pliers.
Vayeta	Baize.
Velas estearinas, de esperma, de cera	Stearine, sperm, wax candles.
Velas, guardabrisas pä	Candle or lamp shades.
Velita	Weather vane.
Ventana	Windows.
Ventiladores pä cafetal	Fans for coffee.
Ventosas y escarificadores pä niños, estuche con juego de	Case with cupping instruments and scarificators for children.
Ventrera	Belly band.
Verde esmeralda ó verdin	Emerald green.
Verdé cardenillo	Green verdigris.
Verde bajo	Light green.
Verdugon	Rib of adze.
Vergas	Iron beams.
Vertedores pä carbon de cocina	Kitchen coal scoops.
Vestidos de señora	Ladies' dresses.
Veta de cañamo	Hempen rope.
Videl ó videt	Bidet pans.
Vidriado, cacerolas vidriadas	Glazed, enamelled stew pans.
Vidrieras	Sashes.
Vidrios planos pä ventana	Plain window panes.
Vidrios de colores	Coloured panes.
Vidrios plancos	Flat panes or slabs of glass.
Vidrios oscuros	Darkened glass panes.
Vidrios pä claraboya	Deck lights.
Vidrios ardientes	Burning-glasses.
Vidrios agorados pä lamparas	Lamp glasses.
Vidrios de postigo pä quitrin	Plated back lights.
Vidrios lotus gravados	Moons lotus engraved.
Vidrios azogados	Silvered sheets for looking-glasses.
Vigornias	Small vices, or bick irons.
Vigornias pä tonelero, pä herrero	Coopers', smiths' bick irons.
Vigornias pä albeitares	Bick irons for veterinary surgeons.
Vinagreras electro plata con 5 pomos ó botellas	Electro-plate cruet stand with 5 bottles.
Vilbrequins (F.)	Braces.
Viñetes grabados	Engraved labels.
Virimboas (P.)	Jews-harps.

Virola, cuchillos con	Knives with caps or ferrules on handles.
Virola	Shoulder (in cutlery.)
Virola	Ring.
Viruticas, limaduras hierro en	Iron shavings for pyrotechnics.
Vis á bois, têtes plates (F.)	Flat head wood screws.
Visagras, see bisagras	
Vista, de mucha	Very showy.
Vista, loza de vista por el color	Earthenware, showy as to colour.
Vocines de platina pā quitrin	Plated hoops.
Voladoras	Fly wheels.
Voladoras piedras	Stone wheels of crushing machines.
Voladora, balcones 4 pies de	Balconies 4 feet wide.
Volante	Fly wheel or balance wheel.
Volante	Gig or chaise.
Votes ò potes	Holders or oil cans.
Vrilles á tonnelier (F.)	Bung borers.
Vrilles (F.)	Gimlets or augers.
Vrilles à douilles ou à tête pointue	Gimlets with socket or spike.
Vuelta, sierras de	Turning saws.
Vuelta cepillos de vuelta par curbas grandes	Turning planes for large curved.

Y

Yeso en piedra	Chalk in lump.
Yesqueros, yesqueritos de platina	Plated tinder boxes.
Yesqueros labrados, con piedra y eslabon	Figured tinder boxes with flint and steel.
Yugo	Yoke.
Yugo, navajas con cabo ò mango y yugo de marfil	Razors with ivory handle and tang.
Yunques de 2 picos acirados	Anvils with 2 bicks, steeled.
Yunquillas	Beading planes.
Yunta de bueyes	Set or yoke of oxen.
Yute	Jute.

Z

Zacate, maquina pā cortar	Chaff cutting machine.
Zaguan, puertas de	Hall doors.
Zaleas pā coches	Undressed sheepskin rugs for coaches.
Zampa picos, zapapicos	Miners' picks, pick axes.
Zapatos de bicerro, suela sencilla	Calfskin shoes, thin soles.
Zapos pā ratas	Rat traps.
Zarazas, colores firmes	Striped cotton prints for shirting, fast colours.
Zarazas	Imperial cambric printed dresses.
Zarazas	Chintz (sometimes).
Zarcillos	Ear rings.
Zateras	Cooking pans.

Zopanda de goma	India rubber banding.
Zopanda de cuero doble	Double leather banding.
Zopanda de cuero sencillo	Single leather banding.
Zurrones	Bags, sacks, or skins.

FINIS.